AIDS in Africa and the Caribbean

AIDS in Africa and the Caribbean

EDITED BY

George C. Bond
John Kreniske
Ida Susser and
Joan Vincent

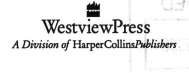

WestviewPress
A Division of HarperCollins*Publishers*

BIE 0850 - 0/2

Copyright © 1997 by Westview Press, A Division of HarperCollins Publishers, Inc.

Published in 1997 in the United States of America by Westview Press, 5500 Central Avenue, Boulder,
Colorado 80301-2877, and in the United Kingdom by Westview Press, 12 Hid's Copse Road, Cum-
nor Hill, Oxford OX2 9JJ

A CIP catalog record for this book is available from the Library of Congress.
ISBN 0-8133-2878-0 (hc)—0-8133-2879-9 (pb)

The paper used in this publication meets the requirements of the American National Standard for
Permanence of Paper for Printed Library Materials Z39.48-1984.

10   9   8   7   6   5   4   3   2   1

Contents

PART THREE
Policy Issues

PART FOUR
Conclusion

Foreword

It is a pleasure to introduce this volume to students of the epidemic of our generation, HIV/AIDS. The authors bring us points of view, observations, and insights that are new and challenging, even to those whose knowledge of the disease already extends well beyond the laboratory and the hospital. Some chapters illustrate anthropologists at work in locales rarely visited by research scientists; others provide ideas and perspectives also rarely visited. Accordingly we believe readers will be stimulated, irked, and in the end, enriched by this book.

Zena Stein

Preface

Most of the essays in this volume, *AIDS in Africa and the Caribbean,* were first given at an international conference on Acquired Immunodeficiency Syndrome (AIDS) in Africa and the Caribbean, co-sponsored by the Institute of African Studies and the HIV Center for Clinical and Behavioral Studies at Columbia University. This was held in New York in November 1991. Professor Zena Stein, the Co-director of the HIV Center, was crucial in organizing the Conference. It was a highly productive gathering of international scholars who considered the theoretical and practical implications of AIDS for African and Caribbean development as well as for the humanities and social sciences.

It was regrettable that many distinguished authorities on the subject were unable to attend, among them Dr. Amana, Dr. Maxine Ankra, Dr. Joseph KiZerbo, the late Dr. Dan Mudoola, and Dr. Christine Obbo. The situation is one of the characteristics of AIDS research in Africa and the Caribbean - the over-commitment of a few scholars whose expertise is sorely needed in so many domains. Papers by the four co-editors have been added to the collection, as well as the subsequently invited papers of Regina McNamara and Maryinez Lyons. Elizabeth Reid generously allowed us to include a paper that advocated placing women at the center of analysis, as well as the paper on development that she presented at the conference.

The AIDS epidemic constitutes a serious challenge for the world today. In 1995, sub-Sahara Africa had by far the largest number of people living with Human Immunodeficiency Virus (HIV), about 13 million, representing around 65% of the world total. Though less than two percent of sub-Sahara's population of 551 million, the known and hidden destructive potential is there. As has been demonstrated time and again, HIV/AIDS knows neither physical nor social boundaries, but follows the paths of human interactions. It is an epidemic that must be viewed in the context of the medical, nutritional, economic, and political conditions of Africa. In immediate terms malnutrition and malaria, for example, are far more severe than AIDS. Civil wars and forms of state and group violence have produced dramatic rates of death among the civilian populations of African countries. Famines, starvation, and refugees are part of the African landscape. The picture may seem to be less grim in the Caribbean, but there too poverty sets the stage for the transmission of HIV.

The very grim features that tend to overshadow and minimize AIDS also provide its context. Thus, in neither Africa nor the Caribbean is the crisis limited to AIDS alone. AIDS should not be treated in isolation or for that matter as a peculiar sociological phenomenon. Rather, it must be dealt with in relation to its historical and social contexts and explored in terms of its consequences for the peoples of Africa and the Caribbean. It is not solely a problem of medicine or an opportunity to apply particular statistical procedures. Research techniques should not be taken as the sum of historical and sociological analysis. For the social scientist there is a real problem that arises with crisis situations such as wars, famines, and epidemics. The problem is how to avoid retreating into anecdotalism and crude journalistic simplifications, as well as hiding behind or reducing human conditions to statistical measures. The challenge lies in integrating crisis situations into sociological and historical analysis as an integral feature of the human condition and an essential element of social theory.

Within the contexts of these major crises, AIDS has demonstrated the limits of our medical abilities and placed in question our 19th century sociological legacies. Confronted with HIV/AIDS, to elicit notions such as society, state, and nation seems arbitrary indeed. To seek explanation in formulations such as "Eurasian," "African," or "Hispanic" structures, as at least one demographer studying AIDS has done, seems bizarre (Tierney *New York Times,* Oct. 19, 1990). Treatment and prevention lie beyond the boundaries of these intellectual and political fabrications and require more precise units of analysis. They point to the necessity of understanding cultural and social processes that frame and yet, transcend the medical moment. There is an explosive temporal and spacial dimension to HIV/AIDS. The virus is not immediately expressed as AIDS and is disseminated along the main pathways of essential human activities. It spreads without being diagnosed by its human carriers.

In society after society the highest rates of infection are among men and women between the ages of 15 and 45. These are potentially the most productive years. They are also the years of greatest geographical mobility. Education has become an essential aspect of prevention, a social constraint on a biological condition and a medical predicament. As yet, there is no cure for AIDS and the decline in the rate of AIDS in Uganda, for example, has been the product of a prolonged, systematic educational campaign on the part of an African government and local and international organizations (McKinley, 1996: 1).

There is the need for scholars and researchers to refine their formulations and for the moment to discard their big notions and their huge comparisons. For once historians and other social scientists have a grand opportunity to explore the appropriateness of their theories, concepts, and methods, to say nothing of themselves and the behavior of others. For the moment science has failed us and positivism and empiricism are put into the balance. But, perhaps, even more important than that, AIDS knows no boundaries. There is no intervening vector; human beings are the carriers. HIV strikes us at the very process of biological and social reproduction, and, thus, at our posterity. Surveys of knowledge, attitude, behavior, and practice are of limited utility when placed in the practical situations of war, famine, and disease. They tell us little about the relation of AIDS to the movements of labor and problems of structural adjustment; they say little about procedures for recovery and rehabilitation. They do not produce accountability and responsibility between governing regimes and the governed. The ruling classes do not have to rely solely on their own local systems of health for medical treatment. The poor are forced, however, to look to local dispensaries and their own meager financial and social resources.

It is significant that HIV/AIDS has followed the routes of trade and commerce, the movement of labor, goods, and services. We are not here concerned with transport and infrastructure, but with that which underlies and produces relations of production and exchange. There is more to AIDS than "truck drivers" and "prostitutes." The spread of AIDS in the Caribbean and in central and southern Africa is no mystery. But what we still know little about are the implications of AIDS for local populations and their productive potential. AIDS has also spread within the contexts of violent struggles for power and is certainly to be found in the ranks of the military. Just how effective is an army whose soldiers have succumbed to AIDS, especially in countries under military rule? Though it knows no boundaries, we think it not incorrect to say that AIDS tends to concentrate among and is forced upon the politically and economically disempowered such as women and children. Much research and attention should be given to these two populations, as well as to the elderly. Whom do they care for and who will care for them in light of AIDS?

The problems of AIDS should force us to look not only at the dying and the immediate circumstances of death, but also to the conditions of the living and their futures. For us many questions remain, such as the relation of AIDS to economic development, its effects on domestic arrangements and the education of children. How will social units manage in the event of loss of personnel? Will AIDS affect local explanations of events and perceptions of human rights? How will international organizations address AIDS in Africa and the Caribbean? These are but some of the questions which are explored in this collection of essays.

It is perhaps necessary to explain why the focus of this volume is AIDS in Africa and the Caribbean. The case studies presented here are not intended to reflect any kind of African diaspora or to postulate an African connection. Rather the concentration on two African and three Caribbean countries is a function of the research interests of the editors as well as a function of their membership in the International Advisory Group of the HIV Center of Columbia University. The cases presented are most certainly not to be taken as in any way representative of the "Third World" in contrast with AIDS in "western" countries. It is the firm conviction of the editors that AIDS must be studied as a global phenomenon. Several of the essays of this volume attest to the significance of travel, tourism, and migration in the transmission of HIV/AIDS.

In comparative terms, migration is the theme that unites the case studies from Puerto Rico, the Dominican Republic, and Cuba in this volume. The global ethnoscape of the 1980's so delicately drawn by Arjun Appadurai (1992) is ripe with the dangers of HIV infection. Migration is, of course, as old as mankind but it has become accelerated since the 1960s when, as the iron grid of colonialism was lifted from so many new nations, the technology of the United States' technical and intellectual imperialism encouraged hegemonic appreciation in young nations and brain drains from old. In the 1980s, asylum seekers, economic migrants, and family reunification accounted for yet another increase in population movement from western Europe. Travellers (defined by the United Nations, the World Health Organization, and the International Organization for Migration as people entering a country for three months or less) became, as far as AIDS control was concerned, a risk/target group.

> People behave differently when they travel.Tourists travel to seek adventure and new experiences, and to make new friends. Sex is certainly part of the attraction. The usual norms of the home environment no longer control behavior, and travellers separated from their families are all at particular risk (De Schryver and Meheus 1990:55).

In 1990 at a conference of the Society for Applied Anthropology held at York University, England, on "Assembling knowledge to address human problems." Bond and Vincent began to delineate the concept of Multiple Contingent Risk or MCR. The risk situations of labor migrants are typical. They tend to live in low cost, unsanitary housing situations; they are subject to unemployment, underemployment, and poverty. They may, as Susser suggests in her chapter in this volume, be separated from partners and families; many may be lonely; most are vulnerable and exploited. Such conditions lead to poor health in general, less access to health services, and a higher incidence of HIV-related risk behaviors. Further, such migrants have less access to HIV education and information. Susser describes HIV being brought to Puerto Rico by migrants returning from New York and New Jersey; Figueroa (1991) similarly reports the first cases being brought to Jamaica by returning migrant farm workers. Drugs and homosexuality in the "First" world contribute to the introduction and spread of heterosexual AIDS in the "Third" world.

The importance of tourism in HIV transmission has been documented for both Africa and the Caribbean, as has proximity to military and naval bases. AIDS is part of the global economy. Furthermore the AIDS pandemic must, we suggest, be related to global trafficking in drugs, international sales of blood, and similar mid-twentieth century transnational developments.

One of the topics that aroused considerable interest at the conference at which these papers were first given is the origin of the AIDS epidemic. The book by Richard and Rosalind Chirimuuta, *AIDS, Africa and Racism,* published in 1987, captured a controversy in full flight. Whether Western scientists and journalists were inadvertently racist in speculating on the origin of the disease in "darkest Africa" is still a matter raised periodically in local African, Caribbean, and African American newspapers. Most recently, Cindy Patton in *Inventing AIDS* observed that Luc Montagne's insistence on claiming that "AIDS began in Africa," despite no valid evidence or critical understanding of the social versus scientific meaning of locating origins, suggests that he is also largely influenced by cultural stereotypes (1990:149). Patton extends the arguments of Richard and Rosalind Chirimuuta. She is concerned to investigate how the Western invention, as she sees it, of Africa as poverty stricken and heterosexual set medical science on what she calls a genocidal course. She has in mind the fact that Phase Three vaccine trials are being carried out in African countries when they would not be carried out in Europe or America. She also deplores the readiness of medical scientists to absorb the early inscription of Slim disease by Ugandan clinicians into their own conception of 'AIDS'. The prevalence of malarial plasmodium in Uganda led thereafter to the recording of many false HIV positive results.

The editors are very aware of a major lack in this volume. We do not intend to marginalize or silence the voices of Africans and persons from the Caribbean, either researchers or AIDS victims. We are very conscious that research in Uganda, for example, could not have been done by the anthropologists and historian whose work you will be reading in this volume, were it not for Ugandans' willingness to share their knowledge and views. The two articles by David Serwadda, the clinician who first diagnosed Slim in 1982, are taken by Bond and Vincent as benchmarks in the history of the AIDS epidemic in Uganda.

In many respects, the study of HIV/AIDS has collapsed the boundaries between researchers and practitioners. The disease transcends parochial concerns and requires cooperation in collecting and disseminating a wide range of information to inform scholarship and policy. This collection of essays is a step in that direction.

George C. Bond
Director, Institute of African Studies

Acknowledgments

The Institute of African Studies wishes to acknowledge and express its gratitude to the HIV Center for its major support in assisting in the funding of the conference. Major funding came from the Center's grant, NIMH 2P50MH43520. We also wish to thank the conference participants, and the African Institute's faculty, students, and staff, all of whom made the conference possible. Special thanks are due to Ms Rand, the African Institute's administrative assistant, and Molly Doane, who worked on the manuscript.

Ida Susser and George C. Bond

PART ONE
Introduction

1

The Anthropology of AIDS in Africa and the Caribbean

George C. Bond, John Kreniske,
Ida Susser, and Joan Vincent

Introduction

This book emerged from discussion among medical anthropologists, anthropologists who had worked in Africa and the Caribbean and researchers in public health. In 1987, we formed the International Advisory Group (IAG) of the HIV Center for Clinical and Behavioral Sciences and began to try to work out how the knowledge and methods of anthropology could be most useful in addressing the HIV pandemic. In 1991, we organized a conference entitled *The Anthropology of Aids in Africa and the Caribbean: the dimensions of an epidemic,* sponsored by the HIV Center and the Institute of African Studies at Columbia University. This edited volume represents some of the papers from that conference, combined with research papers that emerged later from the IAG.

This chapter and the next one by Anne Akeroyd provide an introduction to HIV/AIDS. Dr. Akeroyd's chapter reviews the literature on the social and cultural context of HIV in Africa. Her brilliant critical essay has methodological, conceptual and theoretical material that goes far beyond the African continent. The essay is essential reading for anthropologists and policy makers world wide. Following the introduction, the first section of the book involves a series of case studies, some by anthropologists and some by researchers in public health. Chapters three through five concern HIV in the Caribbean. Chapters six through nine represent case studies from Africa. The second section of the book presents three analyses of policy issues followed by a concluding statement by Shirley Lindenbaum.

No one anthropological approach is privileged. Yet, the overall perspective assumes that political/economic conditions will structure as well as be changed by the development of public health policy, the formation of social movements and the emerging and dissonant discourses around HIV.

We have consciously included ethnographic case studies, analysis of issues by researchers in public health and policy statements and critiques in this edited collection in the effort to demonstrate the necessary interaction between the different areas. Anthropologists have been known to avoid or denigrate research that has immediate policy implications, especially if the work was, in fact, designed to answer policy questions. From the other side, policy analysts have avoided the use of anthropological research and literature, viewing anthropological concepts as too abstract and research procedures as too lengthy to be of use for immediate policy decisions. Both these barriers to the communication and dissemination of information have been breaking down in the past decade. The permeability of the disciplinary walls has been greatly increased in confrontation with the disaster of HIV (National Academy of Sciences 1986; Herdt and Lindenbaum 1992; Fox and Fee 1992;Van de Walle 1990; Singer et al. 1990). It is hoped that the format of this book and the articles collected here will add to the growing interaction and productive debate among policy makers, public health researchers and anthropologists.

Since this project was conceived in 1990, Asia and Eastern Europe have been rapidly acquiring HIV among ever-increasing numbers of their populations. However, since the first poor countries to manifest the HIV epidemic were in Africa and the Caribbean, the epidemic, our questions concerning it and our knowledge of it are further advanced in these areas. Findings in Africa and the Caribbean will assist in addressing problems developing in areas such as Thailand, India and Poland.

The Moving Frontier of HIV Infection

Legacies of colonialism and poverty have combined with the contemporary global economy to worsen the impact of "natural" disasters in both Africa and the Caribbean. Drought and famine have devastated regions of Africa, bringing with them immediate death through epidemics of infectious diseases such as cholera as well as high rates of mortality from malnutrition. Each of these disasters also marks the trail for the "moving frontier" of AIDS as reported by Bond and Vincent in this volume.

Governments with few financial resources are vulnerable to military takeovers, ethnic hostilities and undermining by international intervention, both direct and indirect. Thus, war and instability have exacerbated the risks of HIV infection in Uganda, (as documented by Bond and Vincent in chapter 6) as in many parts of the Third World. Military movements combined with unprecedented shifts of civilian populations, such as the tragic situation in Rwanda and the continuous desperate departure of Haitians from Haiti, all disrupt families, and leave women and children with few options for survival. Such events create prime conditions for the unfettered transmission of the HIV virus, as well as many other diseases and violent forms of death.

Questions Concerning HIV Infection in Third World Countries

HIV is one source of crisis and suffering among many that desperately call for attention. Even in a middle income community in Europe or the United States where people expect to live to old age and cure what diseases they may contract, HIV battles for center stage with other life-threatening diseases. Social movements have been organized to combat patterns of discrimination and stigma associated with the disease and to convince national policy makers and health care providers of the hazard and the enormity of the suffering caused by HIV infection. Even in communities where treatment is insured and comfortable lifestyles affordable, debates concerning the distribution of funds for research and treatment, and the usefulness of early testing and diagnosis and its impact on the quality of daily life, have constituted an ongoing discussion.

In the poorer countries of the world as indeed in poor areas of the United States, the dilemmas of making choices as to the allocation of scarce resources is more extreme. Should HIV take priority over other infectious diseases? Where should these resources come from and who should receive them? If prevention is the only feasible strategy, should funding be devoted to the prevention of HIV alone or to general public health and community health education efforts? Anthropologists and public health researchers and policy makers have to make hard choices. They have to balance their convictions against the requirements of the situation.

Thus, as the case studies in this volume demonstrate, understanding HIV infection in poor countries requires researchers to struggle with a number of issues: such as income inequality, land reform, the alienation of peasants from the land, labor migration, colonial and post-colonial patterns of industrial exploitation, the resulting proliferation of informal settlements, gender hierarchies and the increasing separation of children from their formal family connections. It is only with an understanding of the specific social and historical contexts that an effective mobilization for the prevention of HIV or coping with the devastation of HIV can be implemented (Bond and Vincent 1991a; Susser and Kreniske this volume; Fee and Fox 1992; National Research Council 1989).

Poverty and social disruption force us to evaluate moral issues within a different frame. Questions which appear to lead to one answer in the United States may generate contrasting responses in other situations. Consider simply whether to recommend that a young mother with possible symptoms should be encouraged to seek an HIV test.

Sexual Behavior and Changing
Social Conditions

In Africa, heterosexual sex and its corollary of perinatal transmission is viewed as the major source of HIV transmission. Because of the importance of heterosexual transmission of HIV in Third World countries, medical and public health researchers have focussed on patterns of sexual contact. Anthropological research and methods have been called upon to provide information about changing sexual behavior and expectations among different populations in Africa. While information concerning these issues may be essential for some epidemiological research, anthropologists and other social scientists have been wary of examining data concerning sexual behavior separately from the broader social context in which it was gathered. Research has consistently demonstrated that sexual behavior is conditioned and changed by changing social organization, economic expectations and historical events, even by HIV itself. While sexuality is an important factor in any analysis of HIV transmission, patterns of transmission can only be explained within the broader societal context, such as those analyzed in the case studies presented here.

As Lyons demonstrates in her chapter on the emerging discourse around "African Aids," in Uganda, and as other reviewers have noted, studies purporting to explain the transmission of HIV among different populations by citing such factors as "promiscuity," tend to stigmatize or blame certain groups while failing to explain patterns of transmission (Lyons, this volume; Ankrah 1991; Schoepf 1992b; Van de Walle 1990). Multiple partners alone neither a necessary nor sufficient cause for the transmission of HIV. As Reid's articles and others in this volume demonstrate clearly the social and economic organization within which sexual interactions occur affect the path of the HIV virus.

Cuban Public Health Policy

Two case studies in the first section, on Cuba and Africa, address the issues of HIV from a broad public health perspective. McNamara addresses the issues of STDs and women's access to health care which will be noted below in the discussion of women and HIV. Santana provides an on-the-ground review of the Cuban containment policies and argues that while this may have worked well during a particular period in Cuba, it would be a mistake to conceive of such a policy transplanted to the United States.

Santana's chapter is an important corrective to recent anthropological debates on this issue. She demonstrates the processual development of the Cuban system and shows that while originating as strict containment, policies were forced to change over time as the number of infected people and the lifelong nature of the infection came to be understood. Some of the arguments present in the anthropological literature have neglected the changing nature of the Cuban policies themselves and either suggested that they be adopted (as if unchanging, see Scheper-Hughes 1993) or condemned (also without recognition of their ongoing evolution, see Bolton 1992).

Scheper-Hughes, in her recommendation that Cuban containment policies be considered in the United States, ignores important facets of the Cuban situation which are illuminated by the Santana article. The Cubans who were found to be HIV positive and confined in the sanatoria were treated as an elite with access to televisions, VCR's, air conditioning and good food. They were considered by other Cubans to be living in the height of luxury. Such a policy would be too expensive to maintain were the rates of HIV seropositivity to increase and certainly too expensive to maintain in the United States where even the costs of providing adequate housing for people with AIDS has become a political battle. Thus, the success of the Cuban policy of containment depended partially on the small numbers of infected people, the encompassing and effective public health records and tracking procedures and the life advantages of remaining confined. None of these factors are present in the United States.

Women and HIV Infection

Another major area relating to the prevention and treatment of HIV in poor countries concerns the particular problems of women and HIV and the complex gender hierarchies found in different contexts. This volume raises such issues in the review article by Akeroyd, as well as in several of the case studies, including Susser and Kreniske, McNamara and Reid. As Schoepf (1991), Ankrah (1991) and Reid (this volume) have argued most effectively, women in Third World countries are at an extreme disadvantage in the prevention and treatment of HIV. This is reflected in the growing number of women as opposed to men who are becoming infected. It is similarly reflected in the United States where women becoming infected through heterosexual sex, while still under-represented, constitute the fastest growing group of persons contracting HIV infection.

HIV Infection and Global Travel

HIV exists in a world which has become increasingly global in the movement of both capital and labor. Labor migration to and from the Caribbean to the United States has been a major factor in the migration of HIV infection. Similarly, the development of tourist industries, frequently based on U.S. capital as a replacement for the decline of profits from older colonially established sources such as sugar cane, has also traced the routes for HIV to follow. Kreniske's case study of both labor migration and tourist travel through the Dominican Republic begins to examine the complexities of these different processes within the context of the movement of global capital. He documents the need for Haitian labor on the Dominican sugar plantations and the permanent unofficial settlements of men, women and child migrants who work seasonally in the cane fields. Like many borders crossed by migrant laborers, the borders for HIV are much less well defined than maps and national boundaries imply. Susser and Kreniske's article, connecting experiences in Puerto Rico with the lives of Puerto Rican migrants to the United States adds another dimension to the discussion of the ways in which labor mobility opens the way for HIV.

Santana's description of Cuba within a limited time frame, demonstrates the contrasting policies and experiences reflected in the political differences of the Caribbean islands. While Cuban men and women may or may not differ in their expectations and sexual behavior from people in Puerto Rico and the Dominican Republic, government policies and differing patterns of labor migration and economic dependency have protected Cubans, so far, from the high rates of HIV infection found in other parts of the Caribbean. As political shifts and the disappearance of the polarities of the Cold War open Cuba further to tourism and oscillating labor migration, different issues may quickly emerge.

Policy Issues

The second section of the book includes four articles on policy issues. The first two articles by Reid address two issues central to the conceptualization of policy concerning HIV. She herself spearheaded the AIDS division of the United Nations Development Fund and worked directly with implementing policy. She reorients the perspective of public health workers and development agencies prone to view women with HIV as represented by "prostitutes" or "sex workers." She points out that women at risk for HIV in Africa and elsewhere are, in fact, frequently monogamous, fulfilling the expectations for mothers and wives in a broad spectrum of situations. Since women are at the center of domestic reproduction and sometimes of the household economy as well, the illness and loss of women in their middle years opens entire families to destitution and disintegration. Reid then proceeds to discuss the overall implications for development of an epidemic which devastates the caretakers and economic providers and leaves children and the elderly to work for the future of the society.

The next article, by Rosalind and Richard Chirimuuta, discusses the origin debates around AIDS. In its claims that theories of the origin of AIDS in Africa were inspired more by Western stereotypes than by hard data, it reflects many of the suspicions of people in poor countries as well as African Americans and other groups in the United States. Clearly, this is an important discourse within the HIV literature and must be taken into account in any analysis of the impact of Western medical research on HIV prevention and treatment in Africa and elsewhere.

The last chapter in this section, by Meredeth Turshen, examines early responses by the US Agency for International Development and its subsidiary Family Health International (FHI) to the AIDS epidemic in Africa. Turshen argues that initial reactions involved a misplaced expectation that individual change supported by the provision of condoms and emphasis on safe sex practices would adequately address the overwhelming problems of the new disease. She suggests that attention to broader issues initially would have led to more effective and fundamental prevention and treatment efforts. Many of the issues raised by Turshen have subsequently been taken into account by FHI. This chapter represents an analysis of the forms of discourse and instrumental interventions which appear to come most easily to Western medical practice.

The concluding remarks in the volume were prepared by Shirley Lindenbaum and represent her thoughts based both on the articles in this book and her wide participation in research on HIV infection in the United States and internationally.

2

Sociocultural Aspects of AIDS in Africa: Occupational and Gender Issues

Anne V. Akeroyd

As long as there is widespread poverty, marginalization of risk groups, counter-productive labor practices and denial of women's rights, the fundamental transformation of individuals and societies which is required to ultimately control AIDS in Africa will not occur (Moses and Plummer 1994:127).

Introduction

The HIV/AIDS epidemic continues apace. By late 1994 Africa accounted for a third (34%) of the total reported AIDS cases in adults and children but two-thirds (70%) of the estimated total of global AIDS cases; some three-fifths (over 11 million) of the estimated cumulative global total of HIV-infections in adults; and the 8 million adults estimated to be living with HIV-infection there comprised one half to three-fifths of the worldwide total.[1] Some 700,000 children were born to HIV-positive women in Africa in 1993 alone.[2] Nearly 1 million African children under 5 years are estimated to have been HIV-infected; some 4 million children are expected to be AIDS orphans by the year 2000; in some areas over half the children under 15 years have lost a parent; and the age at which infection occurs is getting lower—currently nearly two thirds of infections are occurring amongst people under 25 years of age.[3] By the year 2000 the World Health Organization expects that some 7.5 million women in Africa could have become infected.[4] The consequences of HIV-infection and AIDS will long continue; but the possibilities for action are limited by stark economic and political realities. As WHO noted, reporting on decisions relating to

AIDS at the 1994 OAU summit meeting in Tunisia, most of the targets set at the 1992 meeting in Dakar had yet to be met.[5] There is broad agreement on the major characteristics of the epidemic in Africa. The clustering of highly affected areas implies that social and geographical contiguity is an important factor in the spread of HIV across boundaries (Pela and Platt 1989:3). Some contributory factors may be cultural, linked especially to patterns of gender relations and subordination of women, and to social and kinship bonds; some are linked to colonial and contemporary political and economic developments (see Zwi and Cabral 1993; Bassett and Mhloyi 1991; Packard 1989; and others are the result of manmade and natural disasters. Marked geographical and socio-spatial differences in seroprevalence rates have been found, with higher rates normally being found in urban populations. Rural areas, though, cannot escape the consequences of the epidemic given the social and economic linkages between rural and urban areas and the movement of people, whether in labor migration areas or not.[6] Even if the incidence of infection is low, rural populations may face a considerable economic and psychological burden, caring for sufferers who return to their rural villages, and/or losing remittances which maintain many rural households and may be critical for socio-economic differentiation.

Heterosexual transmission accounts for over 80% of cases; in Masaka District, Uganda, it now applies to 99% of adult infections (Nunn, Kengeya-Kayondo, Malamba et al. 1994). The small proportion of cases attributed to blood transfusions has been reduced further by safety measures, though practices vary between and within countries. Women and children are commonly said to be more exposed to transfusions than men. Drug abuse should not be overlooked as Pela and Platt (1989) warned. The use of Nigeria, Zambia and now South Africa as international transit routes has increased considerably in the 1990s and inevitably supplies are diverted into the local setting. Though the users of hard drugs have been mostly well-to-do youth currently the appearance of crack cocaine in South African townships is causing considerable concern. The sex ratio of infected people, though varying between age groups and between studies, is generally said to have been approximately equal from the outset. Peak age HIV-prevalence has dropped, especially in women among whom it is generally given as 20-24 years; a high proportion of incident infections is now found in people under 25 years and especially young married women; and there are also more women dying and dying at an earlier age than are men (Decosas and Pedneault 1992:228). The progression to HIV-related conditions and to AIDS seems to be faster in Africa and the time period between diagnosis and death is often short; and a high proportion (up to about 40%) of children born to HIV-infected women will be infected and will die under 5 years. Though these conditions may be a consequence of opportunistic infections and generally poorer ill-health, they may also reflect patient behaviors in presenting later for treatment.

It is not always clear, however, whether the statistics are "artifactual," a reflection of referral practices and gender, socio-economic or occupational biases in access to treatment, of the reliance on pregnant women, STD clinic attenders, and female prostitutes as sentinel populations, or of research practices. Cabral (1993:158), for example, has suggested that one reason why so many people with AIDS needing inpatient care are in referral/teaching hospitals in cities is because senior clinicians welcome the opportunities for research.[7] A striking change in the seroprevalence rate among women in Bangui was attributed to a change in sampling strategy (Mathiot, Lepage, Choaib et al. 1990); and participants may often be restricted to particular age cohorts such as adults aged 15-49. It is also possible that the impact on women is *under*-emphasized: the sex ratio might alter for the worse against women were the African surveillance AIDS case definitions (Bangui, Caracas and Abidjan) to be made gender-sensitive.[8]

Much research into social and sexual contexts of transmission has been driven by the concerns of epidemiology and its emphasis on scapegoated 'risk groups' in monitoring the spread of infection, such as

female prostitutes, "street" youth, and male long-distance truck drivers, miners, military and para-military groups. The commonalities of these disparate groups, such as urban residence, low socioeconomic status, their mobile or transient character, forced segregation of the sexes, and alienation or marginalization, point to some of the social and economic circumstances which underlie risky sexual behavior (Moses and Plummer 1994:126).

However, in areas where prevalence is high, and where "HIV-1 infection has spread well beyond the 'traditional' high risk occupational groups into the general population it is important to look at risk behavior and the social and economic circumstances that determine behavior patterns" (Seeley, Malamba, Nunn et al. 1994:79).

Though this last view also reflects the assumptions of biomedical discourse,[9] it shows an appreciation of external constraints. Indeed, despite their concern with risk "groups," Moses and Plummer emphasize that risk-taking behavior is not solely an individual matter: It is caused ultimately by social and economic factors, and "influencing the underlying causes of the epidemic will do much more to control the spread of HIV infection than the best educational or counseling programmes" (Moses and Plummer 1994:126). Attention to sociocultural aspects and structural factors moves discussion of the problems of transmission away from blaming people for failure to heed warnings. Education *is* important, but heeding and being able to act on advice are complex matters often beyond the control of an individual, as social scientists have long asserted: the argument is indisputable.

Sociocultural and Socioeconomic Aspects

Afflictions and Affections

The tragedy of AIDS strikes not just the individual with the deadly infection, but his or her family and community as well (McGrath, Ankrah, Schumann et al. 1993:56).

The personal, gendered and socio-economic impacts of HIV-related illness and AIDS will vary in different sociocultural and economic systems, between rural and urban areas, between social categories and age cohorts. There will be differences in direct and indirect impacts depending upon the stage of the household developmental cycle, whether the household concerned has a male or female head, and whether it is AIDS-afflicted (households with an ill or deceased member) or AIDS-affected (households for which the death or illness of a family member has meant lost of cash, labor or other support or the addition of orphans) as Barnett and Blaikie (1992) demonstrate.[10] Given the networks within which HIV-infection may spread and the likelihood of multiple cases within a household or extended family, other problems arise. New forms of family structures have arisen in some cases- in Uganda, for example, "children-alone" families (Obbo 1991, cited in Ankrah 1993:18) and grandparent-headed families (Beers et al. 1988, cited in Ankrah 1993:18). The presumption that in Africa the extended family always provides a safety-net has at last been questioned: Seeley, Kajura, Bachengana et al. (1993) found that caring fell primarily on individuals who received only limited support from kin and neighbors.[11] "Care in the community" and "household coping" means mainly care by women: du Guerny and Sjöberg (1993) point out that planners often explicitly or implicitly expect women to shoulder the burden.

As domestic tasks are gender-differentiated male carers may have to take on roles for which they are not well-equipped. Where the epidemic is widespread, as in other disaster situations, eventually there may be too few people to cope financially or domestically (Schopper and Walley 1992; Barnett and Blaikie 1992; McGrath, Ankrah, Schumann et al. 1993; Hunter 1990; Seeley, Wagner, Mulemwa et al. 1991).

Clustering of cases and pockets of infection within families and neighborhoods is to be expected, given the availability and acceptability of people as sexual partners and the restricted networks within which most sexual relations will occur (de Zalduondo, Msamanga and Chen 1989), though little is known in detail about the nature of socio-sexual networks and their ethnic, organizational and religious associations. Obbo has briefly described social and supportive networks in Uganda, showing that there is often "widespread endogamous mating among friends and co-workers" (Obbo 1993b:952). One was a rural network of cultivators, public servants and traders. Two were urban élite networks among members of the salariat in public service and commerce, one (ethnically heterogeneous) based on friendships begun at university and the other (ethnically homogeneous and including some related people) based on secondary school attendance; and these networks were also sex-linked (Obbo 1993a and b).

There are other personal aspects of class, occupational and work-related matters and impacts about which little is published. For example, when housing or housing allowance is provided by the state or commercial employer, a colonial legacy in e.g. Zambia and Malawi, HIV-infected persons who lose their jobs, their spouses, and their children may find themselves homeless. It may well be that some examples of sick or widowed people going back to the rural areas, usually presented as a personal choice, actually arise from lack of choice or from eviction. In the colonial period in central Africa long-term security and welfare provision were ensured by maintaining rural relationships and rights: in the contemporary era of insecurity, so too is the rural safety net vital for many, and coping with HIV/AIDS is no exception.

In general, HIV/AIDS impacts more heavily on the disadvantaged, the poor and the less educated, against whom the balance may be tilted (de Zalduondo, Msamanga and Chen 1989:181). A recent study of socio-economic status and seropositivity in Masaka District, Uganda found three indicators (house type, land holdings and household item index) were inversely associated with seropositivity, and that this held also for spouses and daughters but not sons. However, some indicators such as a permanent brick house might have reflected past rather than current wealth; and the conclusion is cautious:

There is probably no simple association between any one factor of poverty and risk of HIV infection. It is likely, however, that there is a link between an individual's lack of access to resources and the economic strategies adopted to survive and to support a family (Seeley, Malamba, Nunn et al. 1994:87).[12]

Class and Occupational Associations

There is evidence of HIV-infection in people of all social and economic classes, though reports from and about Africa have stressed the impact on élites, the urban educated ruling classes, the bureaucrats, technocrats and businessmen, and have regarded these as particularly at risk. Class and occupational aspects have not been well-researched, and much information is anecdotal or comes from brief reports in the media about, for example, problems of recruitment in the medical sector or deaths in the banking sector. The lack of specificity about personal and socioeconomic details in clinical and epidemiological studies makes well-founded speculation difficult; and, even when women are included in a study, occupational details may not be given by sex (see Nunn, Kengeya-Kayondo, Malamba et al. 1994), or only men's occupations given (Berkley, Widy-Wirski, Okware et al. 1989). Sociological inexactitude in the use of terms like "élite" for waged manual workers also contributes to misapprehension. The social differentials in HIV/AIDS infection, seroprevalence rates and survival times are still not fully clear; some of the apparent associations may be doubted; and as more studies appear and as the epidemic spreads so, too, do the patterns and impacts change.

The Masaka District study used six occupational categories for respondents; as most people had two or more occupations, professional occupations were given preference in allocating people to one category. These were: cultivator (also included craft persons and household staff); trader (also included shopkeepers and medical practitioners); teacher (and religious teachers); other salaried workers (e.g. army personnel, police, drivers, office workers); other occupation; and no employment. The seropositivity rate was 25% for 'other salaried workers'; for other categories the range was 3.7-8.3% with teachers and the unemployed displaying the lowest rates

(Nunn, Kengeya-Kayondo, Malamba et al. 1994). Higher seroprevalence rates among urban dwellers were found in a study of seropositivity among 5690 pregnant women in a mostly rural area within 25 km of Butare in southern Rwanda from in 1989-91. Of the women, 96.4% were farmers, the rest being domestics (1.6%), skilled workers (0.5%) and other (1.5% - housewife, civil servant, vendor and unemployed). For the 528 women who were HIV-seropositive, prevalence among farmers (8.8%) was far below that of domestics (22.5%), skilled workers (24.2%) and other (20.2%). The study also investigated the serostatus of 5171 husbands/partners, 433 of whom were seropositive. Farmers comprised 83.8% of the total; the rest were civil servants (6.6%), skilled workers (6%), drivers (1.2%), merchants (1%), and 1.4% other (day labor, domestic and unemployed) (1%). Male farmers, too, showed the lowest seroprevalence rate (6%); skilled workers (22.3%) and drivers (37.5%) the highest rates (Chao, Bulterys, Musanganire et al. 1994: 372, Table 1). A study of sexual partner changing and condom use of factory workers in Tanzania concluded that information, education and communication (IEC) programs should be expanded beyond commercial sex workers and their clients (Borgdorff, Barongo, Newell et al. 1994).

The impact on the labor force in Zimbabwe has been stressed for several years, and active measures have been taken by employers to provide health education about HIV/AIDS and STDs, the beneficial effects of which are clear (Williams and Ray 1993).[13] Analysis of records of medical aid societies and insurance companies by economists has revealed the socio-economic impact upon the labor force in more detail. Whiteside (1993) examined AIDS deaths of life policy-holders in Zimbabwe from 1986 to end-April 1991. For group life policy holders the three largest categories were general workers (28.3%), clerks (11.2%) and miscellaneous skilled (9.7%), the remainder being mostly skilled workers; among individual policy holders soldiers (38.6%), miscellaneous skilled (17.5%) and teachers (10.5%) headed the list. The average age at death was fairly high, 37.5 years (range 31.4-44.1) for group policy holders and 34.2 years (range 31.1-40.6) for individual holders; almost all were married; and the incidence was higher among mobile people. There are shortcomings in such data (though the companies are now improving their record keeping to facilitate impact analyses) and there are some inherent biases: policy holders are mainly male, and there are differences between those covered by group and by individual policies and by different companies.[14]

Military personnel are a well-known source of STDs, transmitting them in voluntary or coerced unions; and concern about the military as defenders and occupiers and their role in the transmission of HIV is growing. Soldiers may be mobile and at least *de facto* unattached, but they are also relatively affluent and unlike many compatriots may receive a regular cash income (where payment is intermittent weapons facilitate extortion). Military bases are often in rural areas (*pace* Moses and Plummer 1994:126). In Zimbabwe, like other rural growth points, they provide opportunities for commercial sex (Bassett and Mhloyi 1991: 151); and in Namibia sexual networking, especially with local schoolgirls, is spreading HIV-infection into communities around the four bases in the north (Webb 1994).

International peace-keeping operations present particular problems, though Ghana, which is involved in Rwanda, does not send HIV-positive soldiers abroad (Winsbury and Whiteside 1994:4). Senegalese forces get a daily pep talk about safe sex but "soldiers are young, and have a nervous system in their sex."[15] Regular soldiers, however, are captive audiences for safe sex education, guerrillas and insurgents are not. The vulnerability of women and girls in war zones is only too clear: the use of rape as a weapon of war whether by militia or peasants incited by them was widespread in Rwanda (Crary 1995; African Rights 1994). Battle-grounds and peacekeeping zones are obvious "risk situations" (Zwi and Cabral 1993): southern and eastern Africa is no exception.

One male occupational group long singled out as a "risk group" and as the transporter of the virus between communities and countries is lorry drivers or truckers (e.g. Bwayo, Plummer, Omari et al. 1994). However, truckers do not always go casually from prostitute to prostitute: Some of the travelers and traders establish unofficial families along their route, rather like the urban liaisons in South Africa formed by labor migrants. The social problems of migrant and commuter labor and systems are well known, especially of mine labor in South Africa (see Jochelson et al. 1991). New development projects and programs, too, may bring in workers who create a demand for commercial and casual sexual relationships: clients of sex workers in the Gambia included construction workers from South-East and Far-East Asia who were there for some months (Pickering, Todd, Dunn et al. 1992). An interesting suggestion is that HIV impact analyses should be included in planning for these (Decosas and Pedneault 1992, Moses and Plummer 1994:126).

Traders have been heavily implicated (Kaijage 1993; Weiss 1993; Obbo 1993a). Visiting crop buyers were identified by the community in Kagera District, Tanzania as the main external source of danger: they were discouraged from staying on once they had completed their purchases by measures such as shutting down the bars and compensating women who relied on them for a livelihood (de Zalduondo, Msamanga, and Chen 1989). In southern Zambia urban males from neighboring countries, mainly Zaïreans, who deal in *salaula* (second-hand clothing) are scapegoated, but so too are women traders, especially fish-sellers who are believed to engage in promiscuous activities with fishermen so as to get the early fish (Mwale and Burnard 1992).[16] What, too, of the airborne traders in West Africa?

Boeing jets fly to all parts of Angola carrying a dozen politicians, diplomats, bureaucrats and the odd visiting lecturer in the two front rows and a hundred caravaneers and market mammies crowded in behind them . . . In the smaller towns market days are only held on the days when the plane comes in (Birmingham 1989:5).

Will such pilots be accused of carrying a "cloud of death" with them just as Malawian truckers have been blamed for the "highway of death" sweeping down into South Africa? And are there Angolan sex workers traveling round the markets, too, as there are in the Gambia (Pickering, Todd, Dunn et al. 1992), creating yet another link between communities, and urban and rural areas?

Not all men moving within and between countries are truckers and traders, and labor migrants. The clients of Gambian prostitutes in the Medical Research Council project were of varied national origins, were mobile, and were distributed across the class and occupational spectrum. About one third were from the lowest occupational categories, about one-third skilled workers, thirteen percent truck and taxi drivers, nine per cent farmers and eight per cent in white collar and military occupations (Pickering, Todd, Dunn et al. 1992:86). Other mobile people include expatriate consultants, aid workers, pilots, journalists, tourists, businessmen, civil servants, and others: but where are the detailed (let alone repeated) studies of those occupational categories? One neglected category, athletes, has recently been investigated. A study of football, basketball and volleyball teams found that all

> are young adults (18-40 years). They have all the determinants that favor sexual promiscuity: they live for days weeks sometimes months away from their home; they are public stars, so they attract crowds amongst which are many predatory females; they travel a lot . . . they are relatively healthy and wealthy so they can easily afford to have many sexual partners. We were shocked by the amount of casual, hazardous, unprotected and indiscriminant sex in this milieu.[17]

The practitioners of particular occupations singled out as scapegoats are mainly men, their "victims" women. What are the risk factors, the sexual pressures and opportunities in work settings, pressures which may also particularly affect women? Some Zaïrean female entrepreneurs, for example, may be engaged in long distance trade, traveling to West Africa or Europe; that these businesswomen perforce may have to use sexual ploys to get favors, foreign exchange and the like (Schoepf 1992; MacGaffey 1986), is evidence of a sexualized occupational risk. There are few published studies which pay detailed attention to occupational and class issues in respect of women: attention has been directed primarily towards "prostitutes" or "sex workers." "Downmarket" prostitution, women serving a relatively poor clientele, has been emphasized, e.g. in Kenya (Simonsen et al. 1990), and in the Gambia (Pickering, Todd, Dunn et al. 1992)—indeed, the small, expensive high-class prostitution sector catering to the international tourist trade on the Atlantic coast of the Gambia was excluded because it "has little overlap with local life" (ibid: 1992:75), though it would be interesting to know how much power such women have in sexual exchanges compared with their poorer counterparts.[18] The work of Schoepf and others, however, shows how misleading is the constant reiteration of the image of African women as prostitutes and barmaids created by epidemiological studies and the media.[19]

Are "prostitutes" always marginal women? Not invariably so. The Medical Research Council project in the Gambia found that though Gambian sex workers came from low economic status families the Senegalese ones mostly did not. They were better educated than most Gambian women (over one-third had received at least some primary education) though those who worked exclusively in village markets, often traveling in a regular pattern from one to the next, tended to be older, less educated and more often from rural areas (Pickering, Todd, Dunn et al. 1992:82). Even if sex workers are on the fringes of the social settings in which they ply their trade, they have not necessarily been rejected by their families or communities of origin (though it may not always be known or admitted how they earn their living). The Senegalese women in the Gambian project made regular trips home to visit their urban or rural families; accompanying them, the researchers observed that:

> Most enjoyed a higher than average standard of living, . . . The rural families were not impoverished. Their well-being and warm welcome for the visiting daughter proved that she had not faced a dramatic choice of prostitution or poverty (Pickering, Todd, Dunn et al. 1992:79).

Bahaya women from well-off and poor backgrounds have been traveling to urban centers throughout East Africa to practice prostitution since at least the 1930s using their earnings to build houses for themselves and kin, buying land or consumer goods, paying school fees and repaying their bridewealth, et cetera (Kaijage 1993:290-291).[20] Weiss suggests (based on a small sample of 257 marital histories in 1988-90) that about a quarter of Haya women have been involved in activities associated with selling sexual services in urban areas (Weiss 1993:33, n.9); and those who buy land are "purchasing a place of burial and the memorialization it brings with it" (ibid:30). Haya women are only one example of a cross-border flow of women selling sexual services: non-nationals are often heavily involved in the commercial sex trade in Africa (as in other regions of the world) and therefore doubly at risk of being scapegoated.

Ethnic origin may be a factor affecting a woman's choice of sex work or the location in which it is practiced. The MRC Gambian study found that of 248 women only 9% were Gambians: 80% were Senegalese, the rest from elsewhere in West Africa, and most were very mobile, moving around the Senegambian region (Pickering, Todd and Dunn 1992:79). A study in Ethiopia (Duncan, Tibaux, Pelzer et al. 1994) found that Amharas constituted 43% of bargirls, 77% of prostitutes and 58% of *talla* (beer) sellers compared with 26%, 3% and 15% respectively who were Gurage. They suggest this distribution is linked to location, the early age at which Amhara women in lower income groups marry, and that Gurage widows and divorcees are more likely to become traders and merchants, younger rural Amhara women to become bargirls and domestic servants and older ones beer sellers and prostitutes. Although religion (Ethiopian Orthodox) might appear to be significantly associated with prostitution it lost almost all its significance when the ethnic variable was added.[21]

Generalized discussions of "AIDS in Africa" may not be sufficiently sensitive to the differences in women's economic position and power within and between different countries and societies. Probably inevitably, they stress the problems of the poor and pay little attention to middle-class, élite and salaried women, yet HIV-infection among these women may have very important structural consequences in the welfare and educational sectors and, especially in West Africa, the trading sector. In Lesotho, for example, where women occupy a very high proportion of the non-manual jobs, and especially bureaucratic posts, the effects of widespread HIV infection among women would have serious repercussions. Though "élite" women must be put at risk by their husbands' sexual liaisons, their deaths have rarely been singled out for attention (but see Obbo 1993a; Schoepf 1988; and Chao, Bulterys, Musanganire et al. 1994). There are some references to "working women" and women in formal occupations are included in seroprevalence surveys, particularly from Zaïre and the Central African Republic (e.g. Mathiot, Lepage, Choaib et al. 1990; N'Galy, Ryder, Bila et al. 1988). Although in the Masaka District study seropositivity rates in women were somewhat above those for men, no gender breakdown by occupation was provided (Nunn, Kengeya-Kayondo, Malamba et al. 1994), although presumably many women would have been "cultivators." Certainly, in a 1989-1991 study in Butare area, Rwanda almost all the women were farmers (Chao, Bulterys, Musanganire et al. 1994:372, Table 1). Relatively high household income was an important risk factor, but the figures given for monthly income were postulated to be the husband's in the case of high earners (Chao, Bulterys, Musanganire, et al. 1994:379).[22]

Much epidemiological research involves "captive populations," patients or prostitutes attending STD clinics; but reports often provide little social-structural information, other than marital status, as in Keogh, Allen, Almedal and Temahagili's (1994) study of the social impact of HIV infection on women in Kigali, Rwanda. Even when women are categorized by their own occupation other factors may be used to explain seroprevalence rates. A high rate among nurses in Kinshasha was attributed by N'Galy, Ryder, Bila et al. (1988) to the large number of young women in that category, though no information was given about the women (c.6%) who were not nurses, and no explanation was advanced for an even higher rate among male manual workers. The possibility of various types of gender bias in these and other studies needs investigation.[23]

It is thus becoming possible to put together information from scattered sources about occupational hazards and work environments, mainly for men. Too often, though, when an occupation is singled out as a risk factor there is rarely any discussion of *why* that should be so. Most sources are studies which mention the occupations of respondents and participants rather than investigations of particular economic sectors and organizational settings and the risks they pose or facilitate. I turn now to a brief discussion of a particularly salient occupational context, the medical and welfare sector.

Occupational Issues in the Medical Sector

Medical and health workers, male and female, are in key occupations for coping with HIV/AIDS and its associated manifestations, and their responses bring into play work-related issues, cultural beliefs and practices, and gender issues, though they have received surprisingly little attention. The stress of working in hospitals where more than half the patients may not recover seems not to have not been researched, though there are anecdotes about burnout (cf. Barbour 1994). The burden may be exacerbated by admissions policies favoring AIDS patients, and many urban patients, too, may look to hospitals for support when relatives are unable or unwilling to provide help (Cabral 1993:158). There is anecdotal evidence about problems for health personnel; changes in surgical practices (Bayley 1990), and a reluctance to perform operations or post-mortems; and a pilot study in Zambia is investigating mortality among female nurses (Buve, Foster, Mbwili et al. 1994).

Descriptions of the stigmatizing effects of HIV/AIDS on sufferers and their families and the discriminatory behaviors of neighbors, relatives, acquaintances and strangers alike (e.g. Seeley, Kajura, Bachengana et al. 1993; Mcgrath, Ankrah, Schumann et al. 1993) raise questions about the impact upon medical workers ("stigma halo"). What have been the effects on recruitment of doctors and other professional staff and, particularly nursing, which is a major formal sector opportunities for women (or in Mozambique, males)?[24] How have young women in e.g. Zaïre responded to studies showing high seroprevalence rates among nurses? Has nursing come to be seen as an undesirable occupation, or nurses undesirable as sexual partners and wives? Investigation of sexual relationships between hospital staff might also illuminate some epidemiological findings. For example, high rates of infection among nurses in Kinshasha (N'Galy, Ryder, Bila et al. 1988) were attributed to their young age, and no linkage was made with the rates found among the higher level professional medical staff and manual workers; and the researchers did not ask questions about sex in order to make the study acceptable (N'Galy, Ryder, Bila, et al. 1988:1124). Might social network analysis have found intra-hospital socio-sexual circuits were involved in the transmission of HIV? — a Zairean nurse faced sexual pressures from doctors in her clinic (Schoepf 1993).[25]

The brunt of caring for the sick is carried out by women, as carers, nurses, midwives and health workers in hospitals and in the community. Evidence of workplace-related fears, particularly of contagion, has been found among nurses in Zimbabwe (Munodawafa, Bower and Webb 1993), Zambia (Nkowane 1993), Nigeria (Adegboye 1994), Tanzania (Kohi and Horrocks 1994) and elsewhere. How do the nurses now react towards patients with HIV/AIDS? After all,"Tanzanian nurses whose major source of knowledge is still public sources have retained the same cultural and religious views as the society at large" (Kohi and Horrocks 1994:83).

An earlier study of Zambian nurses showed how their practices reflected beliefs in causation which ran counter to the assumptions of western medicine, and that cultural assumptions and value judgements were involved in their attitudes towards and interactions with patients. "Some antagonism in nurse-patient relations comes from cultural concepts of illness," observed Schuster (1981:90). An investigation of midwife-patient interactions in Niamy, Niger by Jaffre and Prual (1994) illuminates the cultural contexts of such behaviors. Technical constraints forced midwives to breach cultural practices and social rules, such as linguistic taboos on using terms related to sexuality which only members of specific "inferior castes" can use; and medical training and scientific discourse have the effect of removing patients from their social frameworks which affected nursing behaviors. Thus,"moral canons are not applied any longer and patients 'lose' their social identity. In this process, they 'lose' also their right to be respected and to be taken care of" (Jaffre and Prual 1994:1072). One example of denial of rights and respect comes from the University Teaching Hospitals' Complex in Ile-Ife, S. Nigeria. A patient was neglected by doctors, nurses and other workers when her HIV status was confirmed, and "a number of other hospital workers only came 'to look at the AIDS patient'" (Adegboye 1994).

In Zambia, Tanzania, Uganda and Malawi much home and community care is supervised by nurses or midwives.[26] In Kgatleng District, Botswana a program for home-based care of people with HIV/AIDS required Advisory Nurses who work in local clinics to add this task to their normal case load. Though the nurses interviewed were positive about the AIDS program seven out of the nine admitted to finding the work difficult and depressing, partly because of the nature of AIDS-related issues, especially the need to discuss emotions and sexual issues, and partly because of work-related issues such as the new and demanding task of contact tracing and lack of a safe place to keep records (Buwalda, Kruijthoff, de Bruyn and Hogewoning 1993).

Even in hospitals, however, much of the daily care is given by relatives, mainly women. In the University Teaching Hospital, Lusaka, Zambia nurses played an impersonal role, spent little time with patients, providing only medications and routine nursing care, whereas relatives when present did most of the nursing care such as bathing and feeding (Nkowane 1993). Women (average age 42 years) comprised 75% of 150 "helpers" looking after inpatients (not all people with AIDS) interviewed by Foster (1993) in Monze District Hospital, Zambia. Most of them were farmers, which had implications for maize production. A nationally famous Salvation Army hospital in S. Zambia which attracted AIDS patients from all over the country provided a sleeping shelter and toilet facilities (though not food or firewood) for relatives, some of whom had to stay for two or three months. Women who had brought sick or dying relatives (mostly husbands or daughters) might themselves become the focus of fears: People living near the hospital suggested that they were thought to establish liaisons with local men in order to survive when funds ran out (Mwale and Bernard 1992:36).

Another issue related to professional conduct is attitudes towards medical confidentiality and openness about HIV status. The discussions have been complicated by claims and counterclaims about secrecy, confidentiality and privacy in African cultural systems. These matters have now begun to be discussed more widely, particularly as concern has grown about discrimination in the workplace and the community (Danziger 1994), and the likelihood that sick people and their kin will be stigmatized. Because of this, and as a consequence of the development of counseling services, confidentiality is now being urged (Lie and Biswalo 1994; Buwalda, Kruijthoff, de Bruyn and Hogewoning 1994).[27]

Anthropologists would expect to find causal factors such as witchcraft and sorcery, spirit possession, the ancestors, luck, God and the like adduced to explain *why* people have been infected and, especially, why those who *should* be vulnerable (judging by their behaviors) are apparently invulnerable. When such reasons are advanced by respondents in KABP surveys, even by those who also demonstrate "correct" knowledge of the transmission modes for HIV, they tend to be treated as evidence of faulty knowledge, mistakes, ignorance or superstition. Is this but a public stance, one deemed appropriate for the scientific journal? Might such views be the very stuff of informal accounts, gossip and personal fears among doctors and other medical personnel? Are medical specialists trained in scientific western medicine reluctant to grant credence or validity to "traditional" views held by their patients? What is the effect of a constant flow of expatriate medical specialists and researchers who may well regard such beliefs as superstition? Understanding emic concepts, their bases in cultural concepts, religious doctrines and gendered discourses, and their role in aetiology, health care and risk prevention, is crucial, though there are few publications relating to HIV/AIDS (in contrast to other diseases). Traditional healers have received attention, mainly because of their potential preventative role (e.g. Green, Dokwe and Dupree 1995; Green, Jurg and Dgedge 1993; Ingstad 1990), but also because of the numbers of people who have recourse to them, often paying considerable sums for treatment and traveling long distances to seek help. But there is little about the fears, beliefs, attitudes and practices of medical staff in the formal sector: this is yet another gap in the contextual knowledge needed fully to comprehend the impact and meaning of HIV/AIDS.

The Gender Issue: Problems for Women

Paradoxically, even carers in Southern Zambia may be thought to present a risk to the local community, forced to engage in "dangerous" behaviors in order to acquire their daily wherewithal (Mwale and Burnard 1992). The local explanation for the finding that unmarried daughters in poor households in Masaka District, Uganda were at risk of HIV-infection was that fathers appropriated daughters' earnings so that to get consumer goods these women had to engage in sexual exchanges (Seeley, Malamba, Nunn et al. 1994). Here we have further demonstrations of the significance of gender, more particularly of being female. The relative economic, personal and social vulnerability of women has been well-documented (e.g. Romero-Daza 1994; Obbo 1993a; Schoepf 1993, 1992, 1988; Mcgrath, Schumann, Pearson-Marks et al. 1992; Bassett and Mhloyi 1991; Heise and Elias 1995). Its salience for the transmission of HIV is brought out by studies which situate the sexual act, personal relations and economic strategies in the wider context, such that "linking the macro-level political economy to micro-level ethnography shows how women's survival strategies have turned into death strategies" (Schoepf 1992:279).

This is exemplified by Weiss's (1993) exegesis of a commonplace remark in Buhaya—"A woman . . . she thinks she's getting rich. Goodness! She's buying her grave"—which shows how sexuality, the spread of a fatal disease, economic ambitions and fortunes are inter-connected, and why women's relation to money assumes a symbolic and moral load of their imputed culpability for the spread of AIDS.

Women are still legal minors in many countries or have only recently been granted full adult status[28] and the personal, social, political and economic concomitants of this may be critical in understanding the impact of HIV/AIDS. Their position under customary law is often unfavorable; and even where they are married in accordance with statute law they may still have their personal property removed by a deceased husband's heirs. In sociocultural systems where marriage leads to the severance of natal ties or where women's limited control over resources in cash or kind force them into breaching the norms of support and reciprocity widowhood may make a woman's position additionally precarious. Her chances of remarriage may be slight, especially if she has been blamed for the death, as in Uganda (Obbo 1993a and b; Seeley, Kajura, Bachengana et al. 1993) and Zaïre (Schoepf 1992:272-274). The death of children may adversely affect her access to child labor power, and affect her future welfare. Where resources are scarce it may be girls who are kept out of school, which will affect their future economic prospects. AIDS orphans (see Hunter 1990) may similarly be disadvantaged, and again girls may be more at risk of domestic exploitation or neglect. In Kigali, Rwanda girls were less likely than boys to be in orphanages as they were useful in the house, would bring in bridewealth and could not inherit property, whereas boys were seen as more difficult to educate and less tolerant of authority (Rwandan Red Cross 1992:20-21). Men of all ages may seek young girls as wives or sexual partners to reduce their chances of infection; and there are accounts from various countries of schoolgirls being the target of such attention. The burden of caring may fall more heavily on women, and they may also be forced further into dependency.

The productivity and welfare of female-headed households may suffer, especially where male labor power is necessary in some stages of the agricultural cycle or where male migrants' earnings provide vital support. In much of southern Africa 20-50% of households may have female-heads and a very high proportion of all women may live in rural areas. A women rarely holds land in her own right; and if her relationship with the male landholder is severed her position, and perhaps also of her children, is likely to be precarious. In settlement and tenancy schemes there is often no provision made for women to be tenants or landholders or for the land rights to be transferred to heirs. Pro-natalism is encouraged by tenure and tenancy conditions on development and settlement schemes and in small-scale commercial farming in southern Africa where expansion often depends upon the unpaid or lowly paid labor of (polygamous) wives and children. If the association found in Masaka District holds more widely then female dependents elsewhere might also be at greater risk of infection. The different economic and social consequences of male and female deaths from HIV/AIDS under these conditions have yet to be researched.[29]

Issues of transmission risks and of women's health in the context of AIDS should entail consideration of matters such as rape, child abuse and abortion, as well as circumcision and other cultural forms of violence to the body that may facilitate the transmission of HIV, but there is surprisingly little discussion of these. The sexual abuse of women (and of street children, boys included)[30] is widespread, partly linked to cultural assumptions about relations between men and women and the subordinate (personal and often legal) status of women, partly to the level of violence in the wider society. "Risk situations" are omnipresent for women: In southern Africa in the rural areas, in townships, in schools and universities, refugee camps and war zones, they are raped and abused. These topics are not only under-discussed and under-researched in general; they are rarely, if at all, included among the "risk factors" investigated by clinicians whose focus on "promiscuity" ("paid sex"), in conjunction with their normative model of conjugal and family relations, seems to have precluded attention to them.[31]

The stress laid on condoms in preventing HIV transmission has produced accounts of problems such as cost, unreliability, lack of availability, fears about use, and their unpopularity with either or both sexes.[32] Men do use them; but women face considerable difficulties in insisting on their use. Cultural constraints surrounding condom promotion and use, on who may discuss sexual matters with whom and who should provide sex education, arise frequently when sexuality and AIDS prevention measures are discussed. Less often mentioned are legal, cultural or customary practices, often a legacy of colonialism, which may restrict women's access to contraceptives. Clinics may restrict contraception to married couples on religious and/or legal grounds or require a woman to provide evidence of her husband's permission, as was the case in Swaziland (Armstrong 1987:378-9).[33] Though accounts of the economic and interpersonal problems associated with expecting women to be responsible for men's sexual behavior are common, the complex and crucial issues arising from such laws and practices and the problems they pose are often not adequately addressed. Recent evidence of HIV-infection in young women in a stable (usually married) relationship serves to emphasize this problem. In Butare district, Rwanda, 14.2% of women who had STDs within three years of the study had only had sexual relations in the previous five years with a husband or regular partner (Chao, Bulterys, Musanganire et al. 1994: 374, fig.1). A study in an Ethiopian city found only 9% of women still married to their first husband had no serological evidence of STDs (Duncan, Tibaux, Pelzer et al. 1994:328). Increasingly, researchers emphasize that the onus is on men to take responsibility for the prevention of STD transmission (e.g. Duncan, Tibaux, Pelzer, et al. 1994:332), or that men should regard faithfulness as a reason to boast (Vos 1994:202). Such studies confirm accounts of the powerlessness of women in conjugal and regular sexual relationships to safeguard themselves from the consequences of their partner's extra-marital relationships or other marriages in polygamous unions—or, indeed, from risks in their own sexual liaisons. That there are, though, problems in referring to "Africa" in this respect (as in others)[34] is shown by the degree of control Yoruba women have over their male partners (Orubuloye, Caldwell, and Caldwell 1993).

Though there are many references to men's sexual behavior, their multiple liaisons and the like, there are very few detailed studies of the contextual constraints on male behavior, and how men, masculinity and male sexuality are constructed. A rare, and important contribution is Shire's (1994) semi-autobiographical account of masculinities in Zimbabwe. Developments in this field would help to move the debate forward, by focusing "on women in their social relations with men, on gender relations, and on men as gendered beings or, as Obbo (1993a) puts it: 'HIV transmission: men are the solution'" (Akeroyd 1994b:181).

Sharing the blame and the responsibility between the sexes, could help redress situations as in Uganda where accounts often take a male perspective and where "[i]n general there is widespread insensitivity to women's concerns or suffering" (Obbo 1993a:230). Above all what is needed is the empowerment of women. The vulnerability of women and the need to improve their position (already on the international agenda as an issue in its own right) is now also seen as closely linked to the vulnerability of children to HIV/AIDS (a connection made by African leaders at the 1994 OAU summit meeting). The sharp increase in HIV infections and AIDS cases in women, and their growing burden of caring for others, has now placed them at the center of international concern.[35]

Conclusion: Towards a New Social Agenda— Signs of the Changing Times

At the start of the decade, I drew attention to the numerous and glaring gaps in our knowledge about socio-cultural and other matters.[36] Much research on the social and behavioral aspects in Africa was determined by the AIDS "Mark I" agenda, *"How is HIV transmitted? What is the pattern of sexual relationships? How can people be influenced to change their behavior?"*, and the newer priority areas for research established by the Global Program on AIDS's Social and Behavioral Research Unit of *risk behaviors, explanatory models, and coping responses.* These agendas reflected the interests of biomedical researchers, epidemiological paradigms, and the dominance of the GPA in setting priorities. The range of subjects investigated was accordingly limited, though political and economic factors may partly have been implicated. That social scientists too often were relegated to the role of 'data-producers' rather than taking the lead in setting the research agendas also constrained knowledge about the contemporary socio-economic and personal impacts as well as the long-term potential consequences of HIV/AIDS. There were, and still are, important issues to be considered beyond those involved in transmission, or with alleviating the immediate and short-term consequences of HIV/AIDS for those afflicted and their families, dependents and associates. Another aspect with ethical and methodological as well as substantive consequences was the limited range of perspectives; generally in short supply were: indigenous and participants' perspectives, woman-centered/feminist/non-sexist perspectives, health care professionals' perspectives, and community-based research, and qualitative studies. The impression given by much of the earlier literature on Africa was of a top-down AIDS research world, one in which people were researched *on* rather than *with*, in which research was *of and about* rather than *for* the people being studied; and which followed "a narrowly defined path which excludes from vision the lived experience of most Africans" (Packard 1989:10). The people's voices, especially of those most affected by HIV and AIDS, were almost always silent (literally) or silenced by science; their knowledge, perceptions, interests and concerns did not appear (or not to any great extent) to have informed the research procedures, questions or analyses. There *were* exceptions, the exemplars showing the difference an anthropological approach could make were beginning to appear, studies which took cognizance of the actors' perceptions and views, and also of issues such as structural adjustment, labor migration, urban unemployment, famine and warfare, etc. as the contexts within which HIV will be transmitted and must be studied.

I argued in 1990 for an even broader AIDS "Mark II" agenda, for social scientists to engage in forward, and independent rather than reactive, thinking; to identify possible medium and long-term social, demographic, economic and other consequences, make links with other substantive fields in their disciplines and to engage in reflective and critical thinking. The situation has changed markedly in the first half of the 1990s. The range of approaches has widened, the increasing focus on women, the greater involvement of national researchers, the use of a greater variety of research methods, especially qualitative approaches, have all added to our knowledge. Some of the results have been discussed here, in their own right or to draw attention to gaps in the assessment of the impact of HIV/AIDS upon individuals, families, communities, and organizations. Widening further the research agenda would bring new methods, techniques and disciplines into play in Africa, as it has elsewhere; and there are signs that this is happening. This should, though, also entail attention to the concerns of national researchers and of the people and social units directly and indirectly affected by HIV/AIDS. A paper such as this may draw attention to what we know, and ask *"What do we know about X?"* and *"What else should we be studying?"*; but it should also ask *"For what and for whom are we researching?"* The epidemic is being documented: but we should still ask, *"Whose are the texts which are constructed?"*

Notes

1. World Health Organization. "The current global situation of the HIV/AIDS pandemic as of 31 December 1994," figures 1-3 (Document located at URL: http://gpawww.who.ch/aidscase/current.htm).

2. WHO, "World AIDS Day on 1 December: "AIDS and the family,'" Press Release WHO/92, 29 November 1994.

3.   WHO, "African leaders back OAU call to save children from AIDS," Global AIDSNews, 1994, no.3. The problems of the young and the need to enable them to protect themselves against HIV-infection were recognized in the pledge by the 1994 OAU summit meeting to address the issue of the Child in Africa. Little is known about adolescents and sexuality, and that mostly from KAP surveys.

4.   "HIV infections in Africa reach a total of 10 million, says the WHO," AIDS Analysis Africa 4(1):4.

5.   WHO, "African leaders back OAU call to save children from AIDS," Global AIDSNews, 1994, no.3.

6.   In Igbo-Ora, a rural town about 150 km from Lagos, 82% of 377 adults had visited Lagos within six months of the study, and half of these, including married people, had sexual partners there (Ososanya and Brieger 1994).

7.   There are references to the 'untypicality' of hospital patients, but little information is available—there are studies of referral systems, choices of medical treatment, type of healer etc. but not in relation to HIV/AIDS. Other factors include the provision of home-based care (often favored because of its presumed low cost to the health services) and the selectivity in insurance cover for employees and their families.

8.   In Zambia cervical cancer with advanced tumors increasingly appeared in younger women and death often occurred in under a year from diagnosis, breast cancer was more aggressive in HIV-infected women, and gynecological sepsis was much more common and its outcome worse (Bayley 1990). The three indicator diseases (invasive cervical cancer, tuberculosis, and recurrent pneumonia) added to the CDC's AIDS case definition in 1993 are not fully included in the African definitions; De Cock et al. (1993) suggest adding invasive cervical cancer in their proposed expansion. In the USA attention to gender-related differences in HIV/AIDS, women's health and women's exclusion from medical research and drug trials are now key issues (see Akeroyd 1994a); on these matters in women's health in the Third World see Okojie (1994) and Vlassof (1994).

9.   Reid (1994) shows that current discourse which uses metaphors of epicenters and focuses on core groups involves metaphors of distancing and results in blame and denial, whereas mobilization in affected communities is creating new discourses of inclusion, empowerment and processes which reflect the complexity of the reality of the epidemic. Seidel (1993) identifies one set of discourses as medical, development and medico-moral discourses, and another as legal, human rights, ethical, and activist discourses or, in short, discourses of control or exclusion and discourses of rights and empowerment.

10.   I take AIDS "afflicted" and "affected" from Barnett and Blaikie (1992).

11.   Ankrah suggests reviving the clan and making it the locus of AIDS activity to ensure the family's well-being and continuity, arguing that the clanship system's failure to respond rationally to the menace to its members "may be explained more by the neglect of interveners in their preference for recently introduced models than to a lack of potential of the system to respond" (Ankrah 1993:10). She bases this proposition on old anthropological texts; recent revisionist work suggests anthropologists imposed concepts of clans and lineage structures upon the societies they studied.

12.   This was part of the Medical Research Council (UK) Program on AIDS in Uganda (MRPA) large-scale cohort study of nearly 10,000 people in 15 rural villages with a mainly Baganda population. They used a "wealth ranking" method. The criteria used for selecting household possessions are not given, and though "no interaction was detected between gender and household item index" (Seeley, Malamba, Nunn et al. 1994:82) it looks as though there might have been a bias in favor of men's goods (on gender differences in wealth ranking, see Scoones 1995).

13. "AIDS and the workplace: Signs of hope from Zimbabwe," Global AIDSNews, 1994, no.1, summarizing Williams and Ray (1993).

14. What might be the impact on self-help burial societies, like those in Kgatleng District, Botswana (Brown 1982)? Those societies, mostly formed during the 1970s in response to the adoption of burial in coffins in cemeteries, paid expenses for spouses (at least 90% of members were women) and children of members, and on the death of a member recruited one of the persons covered by that member, usually a daughter to take her or her place.

15. Colonel M'Boup (quoted in Winsbury and Whiteside 1994:4) in a session on the military at the 8th AIDS in Africa Conference, Marrakech, December 1993.

16. On the *salaula* trade see Hansen (1994).

17. Quoted by Winsbury and Whiteside (1994:8) from a poster presentation, "AIDS and Athletes: A Forgotten Group with Risky Behavior," at the 8th AIDS in Africa Conference. Popular musicians, too, have been overlooked, despite their similar lifestyle and the death from AIDS of stars such as the Ugandan, Philly Lutaaya.

18. Though some of the finer differences in behaviors and risks for the women are not given (such as those found elsewhere between street prostitutes, brothel workers and call-girls), this study shows what can be learnt through qualitative research in its descriptions of the links between leisure facilities (bars, dancing, restaurants), other illegal activities (gambling, drug dealing), and the sexual relations between sex workers and other people in these venues.

19. Anthropologists and feminist researchers stress that terms like "prostitute" and "promiscuous" are frequently culturally inappropriate, inaccurate and often offensive (de Zalduondo 1991; Schoepf, 1988, 1992; Standing and Kisekka, 1990). Standing (1992) shows the need to differentiate non-marital/marital/extra-marital/commercial sexual exchanges and to understand them in relation to each other and as part of the exchange spectrum, and argues that only the acquisition of cultural and social knowledge enables the researcher into sexual behavior to formulate "meaningful and sensitive questions."

20. Kaijage (1993) is a rare example of a historically based study; interestingly, he shows continuities in the official responses to STDs.

21. They say a larger study of similar numbers of women in their own cultural environments would be needed to confirm or refute this finding. Given the common association of ethnic group and geographical areas with religious affiliations in sub-Saharan Africa, this association might well hold elsewhere.

22. Apart from problems of estimating cash income in a farming community, the skeptical anthropologist wonders how much the women knew about their husbands' income. Other important risk factors included young age at first pregnancy, low gravidity, cigarette smoking, and history of oral contraceptive use, as well as STDs and multiple sexual partners. This study produced a new and disturbing finding, that male circumcision is a risk factor for *women*, contrary to the more common conclusion that circumcision appears to have a protective effect (Bwayo, Plummer, Omari, et al. 1994; Hunter, Maggwa, Mati et al. 1994).

23. For the impact which a gender aware analysis can make on program planning see du Guerny and Sjöberg (1993).

24. Danziger (1994:909) refers to anecdotal evidence that skilled health workers are moving into the better financed AIDS sector, but does not say where.

25. A pediatric nurse who died recently in Yaounde recorded in her diary the names of over 300 men who had been her lovers since 1982, including doctors in the University Teaching Hospital, important Ministry of Health officials, directors of state corporations. Source: "Beauty who contaminated 300 lovers," New African, February 1994, no.315, p.22.

26. News: "Africa: Nursing is on the Agenda of AIDS Conference," International Nursing Review, July/Aug.1990, 37(4), no.292, p.291.

27. There is concern about the problems that lack of confidentiality about HIV-infection may pose for women, whose position in many communities is precarious. Whether confidentiality can be kept may be a problem: A distinctive vehicle used by a counseling or home-based care service, for example, will reveal the situation to relatives and neighbors.

28. Traditional healers in a focus group study in Zimbabwe claimed that until the 1960s young men and women obeyed the taboo on pre-marital sex, and that the change in behavior was the result of education and the Legal Age of Majority Act (Vos 1994:197)! That Act, enacted in 1982, also made women legal majors, although in many respects they are still not able to exercise full rights.

29. Analogous issues can be found in Barnett and Blaikie (1992) who researched the impact on farming systems in Uganda but they were not concerned with this type of tenure. For an overview of problems facing women farmers see Akeroyd (1991).

30. Street children are open to economic and sexual exploitation in Africa as elsewhere. Numbers have soared in Zimbabwe, many are believed to be HIV-infected, and a social worker has claimed that "many girls from broken homes end up in the city's brothels where the market for young children is increasing as clients become more worried about AIDS" (McIvor 1994). In Uganda "AIDS orphans"have become street children in their communities or nearby towns and survive by petty crime and food thefts (Hunter 1990; also Danziger 1994:911-912).

31. I discuss these issues in Akeroyd (1994c). See also Heise, Raikes, Watts and Zwi (1994), Raikes (1989) and Standing (1992).

32. See, for example, Heise and Elias 1995; Nabaitu, Bachengana and Seeley 1994; Romero-Daza 1994; Obbo 1993a; Schoepf 1988, 1993; McGrath, Schumann, Pearson-Marks et al. 1992; Mwale and Burnard 1992; Bassett and Mhloyi 1991; Kisekka 1990. For an analytic framework of sexuality and power relations see Dixon-Mueller 1993.

33. Armstrong (1987) discusses the problems which minority status and the interaction between and confounding of customary and common law create for Swazi women's access to contraception, abortion, sterilization and health care.

34. See similar comments in Seeley, Kajura, Bachengana et al. (1993) on the "African family."

35. Among the policy principles set out by the European union in its new approach to HIV/AIDS is "gender sensitivity and specificity,"which refers *inter alia* to the need for the political and economic empowerment of women and their legal protection (Dellicour and Fransen 1994:3).

36. In the first version of this paper (some of which is incorporated here), given at the Conference on "AIDS in Africa and the Caribbean: The Documentation of an Epidemic," organized by the Institute of African Studies and the HIV Center, Columbia University, New York, November 5, 1990.

PART TWO
Case Studies

3

AIDS in the
Dominican Republic:
Anthropological Reflections on
the Social Nature of Disease

John Kreniske

Introduction

The AIDS epidemic has been with us since the early 1980s, creeping and sometimes racing, outward from its initial epicenters in America, Europe and Africa. It has displayed an unprecedented ability to sharpen our focus on the most basic realities of culture, class, politics and economics. AIDS has riveted our attention on the fact that there is only one World. Its rich and poor quadrants shade imperceptibly into one another. What hurts one corner of the World ripples outward to the rest.

Despite the fact AIDS is a global problem, it is apparent the burden of the epidemic is not evenly distributed and this balance is increasingly to the disfavor of the poorer, developing nations. It is now estimated that over 700,000 cases of AIDS have occurred in over one hundred and fifty countries. By the turn of the century, there will be five to six million cases. Currently, it is thought that there are at least eight million people carrying the virus worldwide and this number is expected to rise to fifteen to eighteen million by the year 2000.[1] In the developed, industrialized world, the majority of infections are still among men; in the developing world the hammer of AIDS is falling with greatest force on women. Two and a half million women, 80% of the global total of infected women, are to be found in sub-Saharan Africa. Finally, while AIDS itself exacts a terrible toll, the number of infections accompanying AIDS is a factor to contend with. By the year 2010, it is believed that 80% to 90% of all infections will be in developing countries (WH0, June 1990). If we in the developed world are to aid in the control of the epidemic in developing countries, it is necessary that we have some perspective on the way in which the developed and developing worlds have responded to AIDS as well as the conditions in developing countries which modify the course of the epidemic and elicit a socio-medical response.

When the syndrome burst upon the consciousness of the world in 1980 in San Francisco and New York, the initial response, though riddled with confusion and anxiety, was consistent with the main features characteristic of industrialized, technologically advanced, nations. The significant features of the epidemic were rapidly delineated and simultaneously a powerful program of research into the basic nature of the causal agent was begun. The cultural-scientific bias of Western civilization mandated that the response to this new threat would be rapid and technological.

It is now apparent the prospect of a quick "technological fix" from basic science will not materialize. Despite outstanding medical and scientific successes neither prevention nor cure have been achieved; nor will they be soon enough to forestall an international calamity of historic dimensions.

Moreover, as significant as the response of Western science and technology has been, the response in the area of policy and behavioral interventions has been rudderless and feeble (O'Malley 1989). This, too, is consistent with the major features of Western cultures and societies, which, in general, find the natural world more responsive to study and control than the social.

In the "developing world," the experience has, from the first, been different. In those countries of the developing world in which AIDS first appeared, it did not receive the immediate prominence it assumed in the United States and Europe. AIDS took its place among the many deadly epidemic diseases already present. AIDS has yet to displace diarrhea, for example, as a major cause of death. In addition to occurring in environments already stressed by high rates of disease, AIDS is advancing in many societies which for two decades have been in economic decline. These declining social and economic conditions in the developing nations have done much to shape the pattern of the epidemic and the character of the response. In this world, to create or implement a technological response is impossible.

Despite the grim picture presented by developing nations with respect to AIDS and infectious disease, there may be a hopeful paradox emerging in which the leading industrial nations might find the most effective examples of the ways in which to combat HIV infection. In order to examine this possibility, the Dominican Republic will serve as an example of a developing nation confronting the menace of AIDS with few resources other than a clear will to stop the silent destruction of the epidemic.

In its widespread grinding poverty, hunger and disease, the Dominican Republic has much in common with other countries of the developing world where AIDS has already appeared with epidemic force. The dominant features in the consciousness of the people of the Dominican Republic, even as they become aware of the new disease in their midst, are the economic and social realties which antedate AIDS.

This chapter will discuss the impact and progress of the epidemic at two levels. I will first detail some of the significant features of life in the Dominican Republic which form the critical context of the AIDS epidemic. I will then discuss the special circumstances of the sugar worker's camps in the plantations, the *bateyes*, of the Republic. Lastly, I will present an overview of the Dominican response, with some suggestions for the future.

Part One: The Social Context of HIV Infection in the Dominican Republic

In the social study of health and illness, it is fundamental to understand that disease and illness are not random phenomena. Each society by its organization and core economic features produces certain characteristic patterns of disease and death which are specific to it. The load of disease born by each society is, therefore, one indicator of the political economy and social life of that society. Disease, then, is, in large part, a social event expressing the central realities of the society in which it occurs. In what follows, we select several aspects of Dominican society to exemplify the social determinants of the HIV epidemic: poverty, population movements, general health status, health services and sexual behavior. Although these elements are not independent of one another, a separate treatment of each is useful.

Poverty

At the present time, the Dominican Republic is in a state of crisis. Development began to stagnate two decades ago and, since the mid-1980's, the crisis has deepened sharply. This trend is continuing. What this means in terms of daily life is a shortage, for the bulk of the population, of all of the necessities of daily life. Food is a problem for large numbers of people: Milk, cheese and eggs are either scarce, non-existent or priced well beyond the reach of average families. Sugar is produced largely for export and, consequently, is scarce within the Republic. In addition to rising food costs, unemployment is very high—figures of 42% and higher have been published in the Dominican press. Conditions such as these give rise to social tensions which are the collective expression of individual malaise.

There have been both electricity and water riots in various parts of the capital city and around the country. Strikes are common and general strikes have occurred, with some mortality. Yet newspapers still carry accounts of new and deepening privations. Ask anyone on the street about how life is going, and the almost inevitable response will be: "It is too hard. It is just too hard." These conditions render AIDS interventions much more difficult. If people cannot buy food or secure water that is clean enough to wash in—let alone drink—they are not likely to be receptive to messages concerning condom use or the threat of a disease which might kill years from now.

Population Movements. The Dominican Republic comprises two-thirds of the island of Hispaniola in the Caribbean. The economy is based on sugar and tourism, both of which involve differing forms of migration and foreign exchange in the form of dollars brought by tourists and money sent from Dominicans living in the United States. Reliance on the monocropping of sugar for export and the depressed world sugar price are among the factors which have contributed to the current economic crisis besetting the country.

Sugar is grown on large plantations which are heavily dependent on seasonal labor migration from Haiti. As we work our way down the Republic's pyramid of poverty, we find the *bateyes* at its base. Conditions in the camps for the workers are filthy and disease ridden; malnutrition is the rule. Physical abuse is common, and crowding can be intense (Baez 1986; Moya-Pons 1986).

Tourism and the Sex Industry. Beautiful beaches, sunshine, luxury hotels and a robust sex-industry attract visitors from North America, Europe and Japan. It is common for visitors to come to the Dominican Republic (and other islands in the Caribbean) specifically for sex, and sex-tours are organized both in Europe and the United States to facilitate the tourist interested in this type of recreation. In addition to the organized sex-tours and brothels in the Republic, there are less formalized forms of prostitution. One may find congregated at the entrance of the hotels, particularly the foreign hotels, mobs of six and often many more "chulos" (procurers) who offer young women, young boys, "whatever you' d like". On the darkened streets there are boys of varying aggressiveness, pregnant women and grandmothers, all hoping to interest (or coerce) someone, anyone, into paying something for some sort of sexual act. The issue for the sex-minded tourist is not whether sex is available; rather, it is what sort and how much one wishes. The issue for the sex worker is, simply, survival.

In the Dominican Republic, low incomes, and unemployment coupled with inflation—particularly of the prices of essential items—serve as strong motivators for sex work. This is the key to understanding the prevalence of prostitution or sexual work in the country. Poverty, in a country with little or no social welfare, serves as the motive for widespread sexual work. The most highly organized form of sex work is that which is centrally controlled. In this form, the women are kept under strict control and circulated.

There appear to be two circuits in the centralized sex industry, one is circum-Caribbean and the other extends outward to the Middle East and Western Europe. In Amsterdam, a reliable source tells me, Dominican women are in special demand. With regard to the large circuit, the head of an international health agency told me that while they have known of the Caribbean circuit for some time, it is only recently that the agency has become aware of the Middle-East/ Europe circuit. Women are returning home with AIDS. Because it is highly centralized, intervention attempts cannot be directed primarily at the women working in the business. They simply have no say over whether or not they may use preventive measures or safe sex.

In addition to this highly centralized prostitution, there is a less centralized form which is similar to street prostitution in the United States. A *chulo* (procurer) will have one or more women in his employ; he may also have one or two boys assistants who also work sexually for him. There is also "entrepreneurial sex work." The personnel staffing this sector tend to be female but may be male.

While male sex workers may be found virtually anywhere, they tend to concentrate near the tourist areas as "hanky- panky boys" who "date" both male and female tourists. In many areas of the capital, one may find women not only near the hotels but in less predictable locations on the darkened streets. Often, these women work alone or with another women. At times, it would appear they are not engaged in sex work until the moment of the proposition. Their characteristics vary. The lone street worker may be a grandmother, an impoverished pregnant woman, women simply walking down the street who may turn to ask "Do you have a cigarette, do you know the time, do you have five pesos...?"[2]

In the development of interventions for sex workers, it would seem the easiest women to reach will be those who work regularly in sex-work but who are not controlled by a man or an organization. Neither a chulo nor a sexual corporation can be relied upon to be responsive to the risk to their workers; and, since AIDS is a slow virus, they may also disregard the welfare of their clients in as much as many will have difficulty relating their infection to the encounter with their worker. Women working on their own, however, are generally supporting families and have concern for their own and their family's welfare.

Migration

In addition to serving as strong motivation for widespread sex work, poverty and unemployment force many Dominicans to face the rigors of migration to the United States. The requirements for legal migration are stringent and the strictness of these requirements impel many Dominicans to attempt the dangerous passage by "yola" (small open boats) across the Mona Strait to Puerto Rico. One to two thousand Dominicans a year die on this voyage; yet, the number attempting the passage increases yearly. Once they arrive on the shores of Puerto Rico, subjects tell me, and their statements are born out by reports in the Dominican and Puerto Rican press, women are frequently assaulted, usually by private bands of Puerto Ricans and pressed into sex work. It appears from these reports that local police also force Dominican women into sex work, and use the threat of deportation to control the hapless immigrants.

Over a million Dominicans live in the United States, many of them in New York City, where they must live in areas of high HIV prevalence. The forced migration which many Dominicans endure also breaks up family units. Migrants into the United States may be placed at particularly high risk simply by virtue of the areas in which they live and the fact that they are alone. In New York City, there are large numbers of Dominicans living in the Bronx, Washington Heights (Manhattan), and Brooklyn, all areas of high HIV prevalence. It is common for Dominicans to return to the island either when they have amassed sufficient funds to invest in the Dominican Republic or for Navidades (the Christmas-New Year holidays) and men may participate in the consumption of sexual favors on their return. At the present time, there is a possibility that these migrants returning home have contracted the virus in the United States. Nevertheless, those who have contracted the virus in the United States and who do return home for a visit (and they rarely know their HIV status) might be diagnosed on attempting to return to the United States and then refused re-entry—despite the fact they might have acquired the virus in the United States.[3]

The patterns of population movement and the commonness of sexual work in the Republic are determined by the depressed state of the economy which results in the inability of families to pay for food and shelter. It is this poverty which is the underlying determinant of behavior and which stands as an important determinant as well of the rates of HIV in the island. In turn, it is the foci of culture contacts—the resort areas, the ports and the plantations—which are the epicenters of disease transmission. Within the Republic there is also a circulation of people from rural to urban areas and back to the rural village. This provides a clear route of transmission for the virus from areas of high prevalence to areas of low prevalence. No area in the country is protected and we may expect that all areas of the country will experience a growing mortality due to AIDS.

It is not possible to over-emphasize the importance of the circulation of people within the Dominican Republic. It takes on a particularly trenchant character when one considers that in various parts of the countryside a form of serial polygamy exists. By this I mean that in addition to informal liaisons, men who have the means, will progress from one wife to another while maintaining several mistresses.

Sexually Transmitted Diseases and AIDS in the Dominican Republic

Syphilis and gonorrhea rates for the Dominican Republic are thought to be high. In 1986, they were reported to be 178 per 100,000 for syphilis and 157 per 100,000 for gonorrhea. Along routes of travel, however, rates of 50% for STDs among women coming to prenatal clinics are common (Moya, PROCETS, personal communication 1989).

The first case of AIDS in the Dominican Republic was diagnosed in 1985 and by the end of 1986, 136 cases had been confirmed. In July 1985, the Dominican Republic Ministry of Public Health began an aggressive seroepidemiological and psychological AIDS research program in order to provide the basis for preventive action. At that time, they found a point prevalence of HTLV-III of 1.5% among 963 blood donors in 60 blood banks (Guerrero, De Moya and Garip 1985) and in 1986 a 1.4% HIV seroprevalence among 980 sex workers in the five largest cities (Guerrero, De Moya and Garip 1986). In 1987, 2000 seasonal workers in the border ports were found to have an overall prevalence of 3% (Guerrero, Garris and Koenig 1987). The situation is worsening rapidly. There are currently 1,202 cases of AIDS in the Dominican Republic, with a case rate of 17 per 100,000. The rapid growth of the epidemic is indicated by the fact that forty-three percent of cases were reported in 1989 and the pattern is shifting in the direction of heterosexual transmission (53%) with a male-female sex ratio of 2.2:1[4] (Garris et al. 1991). While the epidemic may have started later in the Dominican Republic than in the U.S. and Africa, conditions are comparable with those African countries experiencing the most devastating effects of the epidemic. In addition to foreign travel to high risk areas of the United States, the health care and public health systems of the Republic have virtually collapsed. This bears directly upon ability to report the spread of the epidemic accurately as well as the ability to treat those infected. The public hospitals have been unable to supply care to any degree for several years. There are few if any antibiotics generally available and the health care that is available is of the most primitive kind. This serves as but one indicator of more general conditions which will impel the epidemic to truly disastrous proportions. It is the very difficulty of conditions in the Dominican Republic which makes the response to the deepening epidemic so challenging.

Part Two: The *Batey*

The pockets of sub-populations at greatest risk as the epidemic proceeds are not uniformly represented in the general population. One of these populations is that of cane workers in the Republic's sugar plantations (*bateyes*). This population stands at very high risk because of the conditions under which it exists— though it may be that not all *bateyes* will display the same risk and there is considerable variation with respect to crucial features such as migration.

The *batey* (pl. *bateyes*) are camps in which workers in the sugar industry of the Dominican Republic reside. *Bateyes* may differ on the basis of a number of specific characteristics and one of these is size. They may number only a few hundred or one to two thousand people. While *bateyes* may differ in a number of respects, all *bateyes* are extraordinarily "utilitarian" in character.

In the Dominican literature the society of the *bateyes* has been referred to as "the most brutal and enslaving (esclavizante) in the world" (Moscoso Puello 19:33-34, in Moya-Pons 1986:17). The fundamental rule of *batey* life is that "no one counts for anything" (Moya-Pons et al. 1986:108). Of those workers in the *batey* surveyed in a study sponsored by the Consejo Estatal Azucar (the government owned and operated corporation for the *bateyes*), over sixty percent of workers reported maltreatment ranging from beatings to verbal abuse and humiliation; yet this must be added to the fact that the accident rate in the *bateyes* ranges between 32 and 66 percent (Moya-Pons 1986:319). In many countries where sugar cane is an important crop, workers are provided with steel toed shoes, metal arm protectors and other items to protect them from injury. None of these are supplied in the Dominican Republic and workers tend to work barefoot. Over 75% of the accidents in the *bateyes* occur in the cane and range from cuts of varying severity to amputation of limbs. All of this takes place in a context in which there is a virtual lack of health care, and no guarantee that access will be granted to whatever care might be available.

The Populations of the Bateyes: The Dominican-Haitian Divide

To the outsider, the *bateyes* present a grimly uniform view of poverty, dependence on foreign, Haitian, migration and very poor sanitary and health conditions. However there is considerable micro-variation between *bateyes* both with respect to the quality of life and health conditions. There is also considerable variation in the mix of the population. The number of Dominicans may vary, or the number of Haitians, the number of *kongoeses* (new migrants) or *viejos* (old migrants) may vary considerably. There may also be a transient population of Dominican day-laborers, *arrayanos* (Haitian Dominicans) and *an-bas-fil* (illegal Haitians, also called *agachados*). Significant numbers of both Dominicans and Haitians may remain as permanent residents in or around a *batey*. Migration history and the nature of contacts between a batey and the outside world may emerge as significant components in HIV status for the population.

The population of the *bateyes* tends to be male (56%), young (41 years old or less, and only 9% are 55 years old or older). Sexual relations may begin at around twelve years of age and on the basis of age alone, the greater part of the population of the *bateyes* may stand at risk of AIDS.

For the estimated forty-four percent of the population that is female[5], there are few sources of regular employment. A few women may work doing small jobs in the *batey*. Other than this, the only reliable income for women is sexual work. For the men, cane work represents the only regular income and this is only for six months of the year (all figures from Moya-Pons 1984). During the off season (tiempo muerto) there is little work, less money and very little food. People will forage for edible plants and, when possible, go to the nearest town to buy small quantities of rice and oil. I have been in *bateyes* where, as late afternoon approached, dozens of people would be boiling water in tiny pots outside their huts (*casuchas*). No one had more than a few wild greens to cook and many had nothing but the water they were boiling.

Residents and Categories of Residents (the Old, the Infirm, Women and Children). Though the official population of the *batey* is comprised of largely transient migrant workers, there is a large unofficial and unenumerated population of women, children, and "informal workers," as well as the aged and incapacitated. This population may, in fact, outnumber the registered population. Women stand at high risk because of the necessity of engaging in sexual work. Children stand at risk because of perinatal transmission and the early onset of sexual activity. Women must frequently engage in sexual work because of the migratory character of the male population which is exacerbated by a high male morbidity and mortality from disease and injury. Because of the lack of year round employment for Haitian men, families tend to be of the female headed matrilocal type. They will tend to be generationally shallow and, in view of the limited economic opportunities, they will be fragile. Even men who no longer engage in seasonal migration between Haiti and the Dominican Republic are very likely to find it necessary to move to other locations— often many other locations— to find summer work. This is an aspect of *batey* life which is significant for the social organization and life of the *batey* and for the transmission of HIV into and out of the *bateyes*.

Formal and Informal Political Authority

The formal structure of political power and authority in the *batey* resides in the corporate hierarchy responsible for overseeing the operation of the *batey*. In order to enforce its authority, this body maintains a private armed guard—the *guardia compestre*—and during harvest (*zafra*) it relies upon active support from the local police and military. The informal structure of power in the *batey* is more complex and may include both secular and religious charismatic leaders. Much of the informal authority of the *batey* will be invested in the *Gágá* secret societies, the popular religion of rural Dominicans. A Dominican form of *vodu* is the embodiment of grass roots political-religious power.

There are also informal networks of support and exchange which constitute the skeletal structure around which the dynamics of the community is constructed. Health education and AIDS intervention efforts must be cognizant of the existence and limitations of these networks as channels of communication and sources of legitimation. They must also be aware of the dynamic interaction between formal and informal structures, since this may do much to influence actual conduct and freedom to act within the *batey*.

The Health of the Population: Malnutrition, Mortality, Morbidity

As much as ninety-eight percent of the population in the *batey* may experience protein deficiency as well as "gross calory deficiencies" (Moya-Pons 1986:311). There is a concomitant deficiency of nutrients as well. These deficiencies are estimated to range from 94% of the population deficient for iron to 96% deficient for vitamin A.

Infant and child mortality can be expected to relate to poor nutrition, but because of the conditions of the *bateyes* and the virtual non-existence of health care, infant and child mortality cannot be surveyed directly. It is possible to gain some sense of the situation from household surveys for "the number of children dead." In the *bateyes* of the capital area, researchers found over a third of families surveyed reported one child dead and twenty percent claimed three children dead. The infant and child mortality in the *bateyes* in general must be at least as high. In the South and East, for example, almost fifty percent of families surveyed reported having lost one child and ten percent of families surveyed reported three dead children.

Much of this mortality may be attributed directly or indirectly to malnutrition. Over eighty percent of children in the *bateyes* are breast fed for more than one year. While breast feeding provides adequate nutrition for the first months of life, when children of two to three years of age rely entirely on mother's milk for their nutritional needs, they will suffer from severe malnutrition and anemia. This practice also results in the commonness of the "second child" phenomenon. If a second child is born during the period the first child is nursing, the first child will likely die of malnutrition or a malnutrition-related infectious disease.

There is little systematic epidemiology for the *bateyes*. Few official figures are kept concerning the condition of the population, and though the population is restricted to the *batey* during harvest, it tends to be highly mobile and its composition can change radically in a short period of time. The study of the Consejo Estatal del Azucar (CEA) gives figures to help fill in the "terra incognita" of *batey* life. There are numerous cases of leishmaniasis and malaria in the *bateyes* and these vary with general ecological conditions. The CEA gives a rate of 22% for leprosy, 15% for tuberculosis and 39% for venereal diseases in all *bateyes* (Moya-Pons 1986:314, 317). No rates or percentages are given for other parasitic diseases, but it is quite safe to assume that virtually all inhabitants of the *bateyes* carry one or more parasites.

Despite the commonness of parasitic infections in the Dominican Republic and the *bateyes*, the vast majority (82%) of those questioned in the CEA study did not know the cause of or means of avoiding infection. This lack of knowledge correlates with a fatalism regarding disease and the belief in its magical causation that will be discussed again in dealing with interventions for the bateys. It is one of the critical factors bearing upon the success of any health intervention in this situation.

Consistent with a failure to grasp the naturalistic causes of disease, most inhabitants of the *bateyes* neither seek nor receive medical care. The failure to utilize health care that might be available in some cases is not the fault of the *batey* workers themselves. In order to leave a given *batey* to go to a health post at the *ingenio* (mill), the worker during *zafra* (harvest) must pass through three levels of guards (*guardia compestre,* local police and military) none of whom have any incentive to allow the workers to go to the health post and all of whom have orders to allow no one to leave the area of cutting.

It is difficult to express the reality of the intense crowding, the basic problems with the disposal of excrement and the meaning of the fact that many workers and inhabitants of the *bateyes* may eat only once every two or more days. It is as difficult to conceive of as it is to convey the sense of the tenuousness of life when one is surrounded by people infested with external and internal parasites[6] and multiple infectious diseases from malaria and tuberculosis to leprosy and leishmaniasis. In the final analysis, however, it is these which will determine the mode of intervention in the *bateyes* but also, through the inexorable calculus of infectious disease transmission, the levels of AIDS which will be found there as well.

Sexual Beliefs, Practices, and Sexual Work

Sexual activity commences at an early age (about 12 years) and, in the *bateyes*, sex work is common. Sex work is often conducted in *bateyes* other than the one in which women reside. This may be an important link in HIV transmission between *bateyes* and is, in addition, very significant from a social point of view in understanding social networks and intra/inter *batey* communication. In addition to conducting sex work in the *batey*, women, in those *bateyes* located near towns and tourist centers will conduct their work in or around these places as well; thus, they serve as a conduits for HIV into and out of the *batey*.

The context in which sex for money takes place in the *batey* requires some explanation. The pay received by men does much to determine both the character of sex work and the degree to which it may predispose to the transmission of HIV (and every other sexually transmitted disease). Because cane workers receive minimal salaries, and cannot feel assured they will always, or ever, receive their agreed upon salary, it is not possible for a single man to obtain the services of a woman for the night. It is therefore common for two to several men to pool their money to buy rum and a woman's time. Thus, a single infected man or woman can transmit whatever disease they are carrying almost simultaneously to as many as six to eight other people in a single evening.

In addition to the general practices sketched above, there are also a number of more specific attitudes and beliefs which pertain to sexual behavior and willingness to use condoms. For example, the belief that covering the penis during sexual intercourse is a ridiculous, humorous and unnatural thing to do will certainly bear upon a man's willingness to use a condom. Also, the religion of the *bateyes* is *Gágá* (*vodu*/voodoo); as in many religions there is an identification of life, sex and the sacred. Sex is seen as the expression of the life force and it remains to be determined in what way or to what extent barrier methods may impinge upon this belief.

In addition to bearing directly upon the willingness to use barrier methods of prevention, religion is important in structuring the causal universe of the people. The condom is thought to be irrelevant, for example, because disease is not thought to be produced by external infection. Disease is perceived as part of the fate of an individual arising from within because it has always been present or because of the maleficent magic of a jealous or envious person. Diseases are not transmitted, they arise or are generated. Viewed in this way the condom is singularly inappropriate.

Sexuality and the "Haitian Mystique"

In Dominican folk belief, there is a certain mystique surrounding Haitians, despite the well known hostility between the peoples. Haitians are often seen as having a connection with the past and the primitive which is expressed in their being considered to be more "African" than Dominicans. Connected to this belief is the belief that Haitian men harbor great potency and that many Haitian women possess the "cocomordan" ("biting vagina" or a vagina capable of exerting great pressure). Dominican men deliberately seek out sexual contacts with Haitian women in search of cocomordan. For those who believe in cocomordan, the attraction may override fears of AIDS. In a discussion with a Dominican psychiatrist concerning the belief in cocomordan, he observed that in conducting a study involving Haitian women his assistant decided one of the clients possessed the cocomordan. He declared that he was going to have sex with her and was not dissuaded by the admonition that this woman in particular stood at very high risk of being HIV positive.

Connected to the notion that Haitians are more "African" than Dominicans, they are also thought to be darker than Dominicans. Darkness in both men and women is seen as a quality indicating "strong sexuality". For these reasons, the population of the *bateyes*—though stigmatized—are thought to represent a population of young, virile persons who, in various contexts, will be sought out for the purposes of sexual relations. This adds to their importance as a population for prioritization in the development of interventions.

The idea that Haitians are sexually desirable might contribute to the notion that Haitians living in the Dominican Republic (not recent migrants) may stand at elevated risk of HIV infection. This is given some support by a study of 201 men and 196 women conducted by the Programa Controlar Enfermedades Sexuales y SIDA (PROCETS). Conducting a serosurvey by ethnic origin, PROCETS found that Haitian residents and Haitian Dominicans had rates of 15% and 10% respectively while Haitian immigrants, with a rate of 5%, in 1988, were relatively close to the general Dominican rate of 4% (Capellan and Reyes 1989).

Masísí: Men Who Are Women

Within the *bateyes*, there are men who have been reared as women. They perform women's work and, though they dress as men on most occasions, they will adopt women's dress when "going out" socially. They perform women's work (including bearing water on their head) and relate to men as women. To have sex with *masísí* is thought of as having sex with a woman. It is important to emphasize here that in the view of their fellow inhabitants of the *bateyes*, these men are not simply thought of as women, "ontologically" they **are** women and the external appearance of maleness is quite irrelevant to their true sexuality. *Masísí* conduct themselves as women in almost every way. In addition to performing the household chores of women, they conduct sex work as women and have romances and affairs with men. A *masísí* may marry and in some villages young *masísí* are thought to be particularly troublesome in exercising a magical attraction on married men, who may fall in love with and want to marry them. This is believed to be due to a spell the *masísí* has performed and the wronged wife must in turn perform a rite (which entails smearing menstrual blood on the masísí under specified circumstances) in order to free her husband from the spell. *Masísí* are not only women, but, potentially, very powerful women. From an emic point of view Masisi may be thought of as women; etically they must be considered men.

Religion, Healing, and the Social Order of the Batey

Among the significant residents of the *bateyes* important in shaping our understanding of *batey* culture in implementing interventions are curers (*curiosos* and *curanderos*) and the *houngín* (*vodu* priests). The *houngín* can take on particular significance in the face of a new and difficult to understand disease phenomena such as AIDS. The place of the *houngín* in developing a treatment has been documented for Haiti but remains to be elucidated for the Dominican Republic. There is every reason to believe that the *Gágá* priests will play a similar role in developing a unique etiology and treatment course for AIDS. It is important to intervention efforts to take these individuals into account. Not only can they strongly condition the reception of intervention measures since they provide a framework through which these measures will be understood but, in the face of increasing numbers of deaths, they will be relied upon by local people for cures and explanations. Failing cures, they must find someone to blame. Who they attribute AIDS deaths to and the measures they suggest to remedy the situation can be very important to the intervention and the intervention team.

AIDS and AIDS Interventions in the Bateyes

The prevalence of HIV positivity and AIDS varies considerably between *bateyes*. PROCETS has found an overall seroprevalence of 9% with a 1:1 sex ratio and 59% of the seropositive were at an advanced stage in the progression of the infection (Capellan and Reyes 1989). The lowest rate found in a *batey* was 5% but the highest rate was 25% (Capellan and Reyes 1989). While the male-female ratio is 1:1, a breakdown by age discloses some interesting differences between males and females. Seropositivity begins somewhat higher for men and remains high from the teens into early middle age, but for women the rate peaks in early adulthood (25-34). As mentioned before, sexual activity begins in pre-adolescence and, though we need to gather data on this point, it is possible that boys are more adventurous and active with more partners than girls. The peak for women is relatively late and unlike the males is not bimodal. It occurs, in fact, at a point after which a woman is likely to have born one child or more. This is a period when, even if a man is present, a woman will need additional income for her children to survive. If a man is not present, then there is little alternative but to engage in sex work. This is consistent with what poorer Dominicans and residents of the *bateyes* claim: A woman engages in sex work so that her children will not starve.

Special Risk Factors in the Bateyes. The independent risk factors for HIV positivity in the *bateyes* include a history of chancroid and gonorrhea. Less

Table 3.1 AIDS Diagnoses: *bateyes*, Dominican Republic

			Age in Years	
	15-24	25-34	35-44	45-54
Men	10	8.1	19.4	4.2
Women	7.8	12.0	5.3	0.9

expected is the strong association between trance state and HIV positivity. This association is due to the fact that during Gaga ritual individuals will pass into trance during which they will have sex with multiple partners including same-sex coitus. The individual will likely be aware that sex has taken place though he or she may not be aware of with whom or how often.

Additional risk factors give some support to our general discussion of factors which might be significant. For women, intercourse with foreigners (through sex work) and intercourse with Haitian men in Haiti or the Dominican Republic and bleeding during intercourse were significant. For men, intercourse with Haitian women and intercourse with sex workers emerged as highly significant—though there will be overlap in these categories. It can not be emphasized too often that the higher risk associated with Haitians is not due to their being Haitian per se; rather, it is associated with the socio-economic position of Haitians in the Dominican Republic.

Part Three: Interventions

With HIV infection, intervention is not a question but an imperative. Because effective intervention is an imperative and the epidemic has many unique features, we must examine what is being done, and what could be done with respect to the developing nations of the world. AIDS caught the world by surprise and the international medical network is to be commended for the rapidity with which it turned its skills and methods to gaining an understanding of the extent of the syndrome, and the behaviors contributing to its spread. On the positive side, knowledge was gained rapidly; on the negative side, this knowledge was, and often remains, superficial. This superficiality may be justified by the need for a rapid response. But we are now over a decade into what will be a more or less a permanent epidemic; some reflection on the direction action might take is justified.

In the characterizations I am offering, it should be understood from the outset that I acknowledge much actual variation nationally and internationally—even within the same programs. International AIDS interventions are generally conducted through an indigenous medical establishment. In cooperation with the foreign agency, local populations are contacted. Their knowledge of HIV transmission is ascertained and instruction concerning prevention is given.

From the point of view of anthropology, the significant feature of this is that a local elite represented by well educated and economically better off individuals with a commitment to Western medical methods and conceptualizations is contacting local peoples with whom they may have little culturally or linguistically in common. That is, members of the dominant national group contact members of non-dominant groups and, using the knowledge and authority that pertains to their elite status along with the knowledge and authority derived from foreign counterparts, make demands which are barely comprehensible to the people with whom they are dealing. This is a situation potentially fraught with enormous difficulties; however, experience in population and family planning, for example, has demonstrated that intervention can sometimes be successful.

The limitations inherent in the situation and their implications are much less serious in the case of spreading information concerning birth control and oral rehydration therapy than they are in the case of HIV transmission. These need to be examined. Outstanding among these is the fact that the prevention message is being imposed from outside the community by a group having little in common with the community. The message typically is very specific and targeted to "at risk" individuals and "high risk" behaviors. It will not address the day-to-day concerns of the people—though these may have overwhelming importance for the people themselves. In so far as the message is imparted by outsiders and limited in the issues it addresses, it may be anticipated that only "traces" will remain after the departure of the intervention team.

What is being proposed here is a modification of the traditional model which incorporates or retains much of what has been used in the past, but adds to it. In order to have a coordinated global program, the developed nations must take the lead along with major international agencies such as the United Nations, the World Health Organization and others. In order to have coordinated national programs, the direction must come from central governments and local medical institutions. But a critical element is that local leaders and community groups must be prepared to step forward to help formulate and direct the effort in the most effective and appropriate ways. The point where the model I am offering diverges from the traditional model is the degree to which it attempts to offer a mode of altering behavior within the social structure and concerns of local populations. The guiding assumption is that the degree to which people actively participate will determine success in the long term.

Primary Prevention. The object of primary prevention is to forestall unfavorable health outcomes, whether psychological or physical, by the implementation of strategies at several levels. Primary interventions may aim to (a) modify the environmental surround, (b) remove the agent, e.g. reducing the incidence of HIV through a vaccine program or frequent use of condoms, (c) strengthen the competence of the host population by reinforcing or introducing coping behaviors. Strategies appropriate to HIV intervention in the Dominican Republic must target these three levels for communities and must move to provide social support for HIV positive people. The intervention strategy envisioned here attempts to integrate social and individual levels by connecting HIV social support networks[7] to community level networks addressing more general social concerns.

Competence Building. The effectiveness of intervention strategies in increasing general coping has been demonstrated in several instances in recent times (Slaughter 1983; Berruta-Clement 1984; Pierson et al. 1984; Jordan et al. 1985). Interventions in conditions of poverty for both family functioning and child development have been conducted and demonstrated to be effective over time in the cases of the Houston Parent-Child Development Center Program for Mexican-American children ages 1-3 and their parents and the Headstart Program (Johnson and Breckenridge 1982; Johnson and Walker 1985; Laar and Darlington 1982, Consortium for Longitudinal Studies 1983).

Empowerment. Though beginning with a "top down" approach from the intervention team to the community, the intervention is intended to stimulate activities that will be initiated at the community -level by community groups. In this sense the model being advocated here avoids the paternalism frequently associated with interventions in which professionals take the central, directing roles (Swift 1984). The intervention teams offer assistance based upon community need in order to stimulate community initiated action.

Mutual help and Support Networks. In the United States, one of the potentially most important recent developments has been the explosion of self help groups. Currently, there are over five hundred thousand such groups (Gesten 1987:441). It is significant that these groups have formed in the United States partly as a response to decreasing allocations from the Federal Government for health, increasing health care costs and a general flattening of the economy. The indication from these groups is that individuals with *similar interests* can do much to affect their situation in a positive way. It is significant that most mutual help groups are either autonomous or a mix of professional and non-professional direction (Powell 1985). This is especially important in the context of HIV prevention in formulating interventions for the Dominican Republic and other developing nations inasmuch as efforts must be developed on an unprecedented scale while simultaneously providing support for infected individuals. The scale of these efforts requires decentralization, community involvement and autonomous direction with as little intervention from central authority as might be practicable.

In the view presented here, mutual help groups should be considered distinct from social support groups. Mutual help groups are envisioned as fairly broad-based community groups built up around a core of issues of general concern, e.g., controllable infectious diseases, including HIV, improvement of diet or transport. These are problems of general concern which cut across communities regardless of other interests and affiliations.

Social support groups and social support networks, on the other hand, should be targeted to highly specific problems and interests e.g., support groups for people with AIDS or HIV positives, support groups for orphans of people who have died of AIDS and groups to support families which have lost people to AIDS. The evidence for the effect of social support is strong. There is considerable evidence of its positive effect in aiding coping (Bloom 1985) and in facilitating the activities of informal care givers (Gottlieb 1983) and is particularly appropriate for "groups at risk" (Mitchell et al. 1982).

Conclusion

In this chapter, I have discussed the AIDS epidemic through the case of the Dominican Republic. My intention has been to illustrate the force of those conditions which I consider to be most important in fostering transmission—particularly high rates of transmission. Principle among these is poverty, for poverty delimits and severely structures the choices available to people. People existing under such constraints suffer a feeling of hopelessness which is justified; and, it is this hopelessness against which we must struggle in the first instance if we are to make a positive difference in the epidemic.

There are ironies that beset the study of AIDS both nationally and internationally. For example, the problem of the epidemic, and the many problems which serve to fuel it, are often presented as though there is little that can be done. While little can be done to *remedy* the situation, much can be done to ameliorate it. In fact, because HIV transmission is so deeply social, so closely connected to the basic conditions of life, in attacking the epidemic, it is possible to attack the multiple evils that feed it.

The epidemic can be dealt with; and, the cost of dealing with it could be relatively low. Simultaneously, we would finally be dealing with reducing sexually transmitted disease, reducing malnutrition, reducing infant mortality and slowing population growth. We would be directing efforts into the part of social systems around the world which, in fact, may be most amenable to change. In the process, these social organizations would be reinforced where now, in the most affected areas of the world, they stand in danger of collapsing under the weight of the many human burdens to which it has been subjected. AIDS, as an epidemic, can be stopped. The poverty that feeds it can be alleviated. The ignorance and fear on which it feeds can be dispelled. It simply requires that those who have the power to be most helpful find the decency, charity and political will to act and that those who have been most obstructive step aside.

Notes

1. All figures from WHO June, 1990; the World Health Organization now estimates an upper limit to the epidemic of 40 million cases by 2000. A recent pre-publication article of the new volume by the Harvard International group suggests that this is a vast under-estimate and Jonathan Mann is quoted to the effect that the number of cases may be as high as 110 million. Whether one takes the low or high estimates, the title of the article discussing the Harvard publication is particularly apt: "Researchers Report Much Grimmer AIDS Outlook: Not Enough Money, Not Enough People, Not Much Hope." (New York Times, 6/4/92) I would simply like to suggest that the amount of money that might be required to instill a somewhat amplified level of hope in this situation is relatively small and is a stark comment on the international indifference to the devastation being caused by this epidemic at the policy making level.

2. Five pesos is about 50 cents.

3. The consequences of this can be quite serious. In a case in which I was involved, the Immigration Service was seeking to deny re-entry to a woman who had clearly been infected in the United States, by her husband. To force an HIV positive person to remain in the Republic is a virtual death sentence. Not only are health services not available, but

John Kreniske

confidentiality is not respected and rejection by every source of possible support is assured.

4. The highest concentrations remain around urban tourist areas and some *bateyes*. In the late 1980s, the ratio was 4:1, and this provoked some interest inasmuch as it was midway between the ratios thought typical of Africa (1:1) and the United States (20:1).

5. The actual number of women and children in a *batey* is probably unknown. Since they are not part of the work force they do not, in a sense, exist. It is notoriously easy to lose track of people who do not exist.

6. Bedbugs, lice, fleas are the external parasites; the internal parasites are constituted by everything from the expected bacteria and viruses to a bestiary of round and flat worms.

7. Composed of friends and family of the intervention team.

4

Community Organizing Around HIV Prevention in Rural Puerto Rico

Ida Susser
John Kreniske

Introduction

In this chapter, we will discuss the changing perceptions and conflicting responses of the people of Yabucoa, Puerto Rico to the emergence of HIV infection on the island. In order to do this we must have an appreciation of the HIV situation in Puerto Rico and the principle factors which have propelled transmission. It is often noted that high HIV seropositivity in the Puerto Rican population is due to drug use. There are other factors which, though less obvious, may have been more insidious and powerful in creating the conditions that have resulted in high rates of seropositivity. Among these is poverty which creates an economic environment that makes circulating migration an essential and chronic feature of the social environment.

Puerto Rico, with a population of 3,522,037, has the second highest prevalence of AIDS in the United States. The most systematic figures available concerning the prevalence and incidence of HIV infection in Puerto Rico come from San Juan. Epidemiological estimates from San Juan suggest that 8,900 people have become infected with the HIV virus through intravenous drug use, 2,800 through men having sex with men and 1,600 through heterosexual sex. Roughly 20% of the intravenous drug users are women, and women constitute approximately 80% of those infected with the HIV virus through heterosexual sex (Holberg, 1996). These figures indicate that Puerto Rico is an area with a high prevalence of and incidence of infection for intravenous drug using men. It is clear that women are at a high risk for HIV infection through heterosexual sex and specifically as the partners of intravenous drug using men.

A review of the current research and health services on AIDS/HIV prevention in Puerto Rico reveals that the majority of research and service programs are located in the cities of San Juan, Ponce, Mayaguez and Caguas. As these large cities represent only one third of the island's population, the result is a serious lack of knowledge about the remaining two-thirds of the population of 2,300,000 who live outside of the major metropolitan areas and especially about their needs for preventive services. Thus, using the case of Yabucoa as an example of an under-studied area, this chapter focuses on those aspects of social organization significant for understanding the HIV epidemic, the way in which gender patterns may shape local initiatives, and possible strategies for prevention in rural and semi-rural areas of the island of Puerto Rico.

After discussing the general context of HIV transmission in Puerto Rico, we will describe the changing and conflicting perceptions of HIV infection among different groups in the barrios of Yabucoa, the small municipality on the south coast of the island where we have conducted research intermittently since 1982; and, we will describe the formation of an embryonic community organization which began to meet in 1991. This is followed by an analysis of possible routes of HIV infection which are fostered by the structures of migration and employment in the region. We also note patterns of gender hierarchy which affect transmission of AIDS and efforts to prevent infection. In the last section, we discuss the focus of the community group on teenagers and contrast this with the neglect of possible channels of infection for adults. We suggest reasons why certain topics have been easier for people to raise in public and the limitations this imposes on community based efforts to prevent HIV infection.

In order to understand the risks of transmission, the relationship between the international context of Puerto Rican life and the construction of social life on the island must be addressed. One of the most important aspects of this context is migration— which is at the core of the Puerto Rican political economy. Migration is only one of the most obvious signs of the extreme political-economic dependence which has been structured by the United States in defense of its southern border (Kreniske 1987). This dependent relationship has resulted in the island becoming a site for the location of contaminating industry and the source of a constant flow of cheap labor for the metropolitan centers of the United States (viz. Lewis 1963)[1].

Population movements, whether for war or work, leisure or adventure have always facilitated epidemics. Migration involves discontinuity of adult sexual partnerships and may leave migrants with few local social and emotional supports. Sexually transmitted diseases will flourish under such conditions; HIV is a current example. In Puerto Rico, it is migratory labor patterns that are clearly in large part responsible for the spread of HIV from the United States mainland.

Migration and the Context of HIV Infection

In order to understand the factors influencing HIV transmission, we must discuss labor migration with its concomitant separation of household members. Bearing directly on this is the paucity of real employment opportunities in the barrios and, frequently, anywhere on the island. Until two decades ago, most of the residents of the Yabucoa valley worked on the sugar cane plantations or in the sugar mills, but by 1982 only 13% of the male population was working in sugar-related activities (Susser 1985).

By 1990, there were only two factories in the Yabucoa valley employing male workers—both were U.S. owned. One employed up to 1,000 workers, the second only about 100. Nor were all these jobs necessarily available to local men. Some workers in the factories came from as far away as San Juan. Some men from Yabucoa found factory jobs in Humacao, ten miles away, or beyond Humacao along the new highway leading to San Juan. Until recently, women might find a rare job in the region, as secretary, but more frequently, women took in work for textile firms in San Juan or Caguas (cities twenty to forty miles distant). In the last few years, factories and fast food chains in Humacao have been hiring women at an unprecedented rate. For women and men with education beyond high school it is sometimes possible to obtain jobs in the civil service, in nursing, as laboratory technicians or teachers.

Unemployment is a problem for those with and without college degrees. In 1982, for example, among a sample of sixty-six adult men, fifteen years of age or older, five percent worked seasonally in the cane, eight percent worked seasonally in the sugar mill, twelve percent worked for the Union Carbide plant, thirteen percent were either disabled or retired and thirty three percent classified themselves as unemployed (Susser 1985:565). It must be remembered, however, that seasonal work in a sugar related industry can be as little as six weeks out of the year; furthermore, those employed in craft work or as laborers, also work intermittently. This gives the *barrio* at any one time a realistic rate of unemployment among men that is well over fifty percent. During these same years, 70% of the women described themselves as housewives (*ama de casa*). Only 22% self-identified as "unemployed" (Susser 1985:565). While they demonstrate the lack of employment opportunities, particularly for women, in the early 1980's, these findings also illustrate the gender differentiation in expectations and duties heavily entrenched in the community at that period.

Migration

Considering the extreme level of unemployment in Puerto Rico, it is not surprising migration is a constant feature of the environment. There is a strong pull toward a migratory labor market. Wages in the U.S. tend to be at least twice what is paid for equivalent work in Puerto Rico. This difference applies to factory work as well as professional opportunities such as nursing and teaching. Active recruitment from the mainland United States for factory and agricultural workers is a widespread occurrence. As a result of these conditions, more than half of the adult *barrio Ingenio* inhabitants have lived and worked in the continental United States at some time. Similarly, more than half have relatives living in the continental United States. They generally contact relatives and stay with or near them while they search for employment. Networks can be quite extensive and, for example, one woman we interviewed claimed she had worked in canning factories from northern New York down to Florida and had only recently returned to Ingenio where she lives with her new husband and two stepdaughters. Men and women often travel on their own initiative but also travel to and from the U.S. mainland for jobs prearranged through labor recruiters. The work period is specified and the workers generally return home on schedule. Many barrio Ingenio residents have used this method at one time or another.

When people migrate to look for work, households reorganize. For example, when José planned his short-term labor contract, his wife and four children went to live with her parents in a village in the hills. Their house was left locked up for the duration. When another couple went to Springfield, Massachusetts, in search of work, they took two of their children and left the two youngest behind with their maternal grandmother. At a stroke, nuclear families were transformed into stem and matrilocal families. This household flexibility marks the degree to which migration is a long term feature of life in Puerto Rico. Families may, to a certain extent, function to "insulate" members from the outside world. However, households are periodically "opened" to the outside with members joining the northward moving labor diaspora.

Migration is notoriously bad for health[2] and in the case of Puerto Ricans and other Latino groups coming to the United States for employment, conditions for individual migrants may vary widely. For those coming for brief periods with their transportation to the mainland and back paid, with a "dormitory" provided for living, the stay may be unpleasant but relatively secure. For those coming to stay with relatives, there may be some hazards arising from the poor social conditions of El Barrio in the big city, but their prospects are relatively good. Though they will be exposed to the hazards of life in the city, they will have social and, perhaps, economic support; they will be connected to social networks and the community. But, they will also be exposed to the hazards entailed in living in a poor community in the United States.

The risks of living in the United States can be compounded if the migrant does not have support and connections. John Kreniske has done field work with intravenous drug users (IVDUs) in Newark, New Jersey. While working with both Black and Hispanic male IVDUs, he found a small group of young men who supported their drug habit through commercial sex. Their clients were largely from the financial district in Manhattan and Albany; the group traveled the distance between Albany and Newark in a van and sponsored both gay and straight sex parties. While the group was composed of Latinos, the clientele tended to be exclusively Anglo professionals; and, a member interviewed claimed that as many young women as men from lower Manhattan investment firms came to these parties. These men tended to be monolingual in Spanish and relied on the one or two English speaking members to conduct the parties. The group was made up of Central Americans and Puerto Ricans.

Another group of IVDUs encountered by John Kreniske were also monolingual, but exclusively Puerto Rican. They, like the members of the traveling sex group, had come to the United States looking for work. They had a completely unrealistic idea of what social conditions and employment opportunities might be in the United States; and, on arrival had no family or friends on whom they could rely. Specifically, one young man said he had no way of being prepared for the racism he encountered and that this had been a particularly difficult aspect of his experience in the United States[3]. It contributed, he believes, to his sense of personal alienation and crisis which he blames for his turning to drugs.

Faced with dismal and terribly limited employment opportunities and unable to afford the trip back home, these young men drifted into drug use as much for the company of the other users as the anesthesia of the drugs. But, never secure members of the Puerto Rican community, they found themselves virtual outcasts once they became involved with drugs.[4] Should members of either of these groups find the wherewithal to return to the island their chances of being HIV positive from unprotected sex, contaminated needles or both is very high. It would be reasonable to assume that such groups in Newark, New York City, Boston and other metropolitan centers, may form pools of infection. While the cases cited here stand at one extreme, they highlight the hazards of immigration and the way in which immigration exposes the migrant to severe health risks. In no way should these groups be taken to characterize the Latino population of America's cities. Rather, these groups and groups like them are one small portion of that population on which migration and life have been particularly hard.[5]

Yabucoa, Barrio Ingenio, and HIV

Ida Susser and John Kreniske have conducted research in Yabucoa for periods ranging from four months to two weeks almost every summer for twelve years. Over this period we stayed with several families in two of the barrios in the municipality. We conducted randomized surveys concerning household composition, employment, migration and health in one barrio (Ingenio). We have also become familiar with the leaders and members of several community groups in addition to the large group of people mobilized in the social movement against industrial pollution (the focus of the research begun in 1982).

In our work in Yabucoa between 1987 and 1991, we questioned community activists about their views on HIV prevention and their views about gender roles. We also investigated the impact of the local Pentecostal Church groups and leaders of the local Catholic Church on appropriate behavior for men and women and their views concerning HIV prevention, and attitudes towards the issue of AIDS. Since community organizing can have a significant impact on AIDS prevention in supporting safe sexual practices and in working with drug users, one of our aims has been to understand whether local groups were consciously undertaking such functions. We are also evaluating the extent to which the actions of these groups may bear upon patterns of gender hierarchy. If patterns of gender hierarchy remain entrenched, the ability of women to negotiate safe sex practices with men will be severely restricted.

The Emergence of AIDS as an Issue

As of July 1991, there were 24 reported cases of AIDS in the community of Yabucoa (population 36,483), the small municipality which is the focus of this study. By 1987, AIDS had emerged as an issue on national television and in Yabucoa, it was assumed to be connected with drug addicts and gay men. As one woman, Dolores[6], argued, "we shouldn't go to the public pool—there are too many drug addicts and gay men there and we could get AIDS." By 1991, Dolores and a few other families and residents of Yabucoa were beginning to formulate ways to protect their own adolescent children from HIV and had recognized that stigmatizing groups in the population was not an effective approach to the new epidemic.

Initially, in Yabucoa, reactions to HIV were based on discussions in the media. Few cases appeared in the community. Families did not discuss the problem, and men who were thought to be sick were automatically classified as gay by other people in the barrio. Information from national television stressed needle use and homosexuality as the vectors for HIV and reinforced a categorical stigmatizing approach to the disease. When, in 1987 and 1988 we asked people in the barrio about their perceptions of HIV infection, answers ranged from "its only drug addicts and homosexuals," to "I know a man in the barrio who came back to live with his family and seems very sick. He was a nurse and I think he was gay but nobody talks about it." Consistently, answers expressed alienation from and a categorical approach to people with HIV or even the possibility of infection.

By 1990, at least two diverging perspectives on HIV had emerged. Many members of the Pentecostal church associated the spread of HIV with sin and saw HIV infection as punishment for immoral acts. Only children who had been infected perinatally were absolved from this judgement. Among this group, stigmatization of categories such as "homosexuals" and "drug users" continued unabated. In extensive conversations with Juanita, an active Pentecostal, these opinions were expressed repeatedly. When we asked her about her views of people contracting HIV through heterosexual sex, even with a husband or wife, she remained adamant that the problem was previous "immoral" behavior. She insisted that if individuals followed religious precepts, avoided drugs and never practiced sex outside marriage no preventive interventions would be necessary. If they did not follow such rules, in her opinion, they deserved to be punished, even by death.

Juanita's husband, who had also led the environmental movement and later joined the Pentecostal Church, was more flexible in his views. Although not active in HIV prevention in the barrio, he was willing to consider the need to develop community prevention programs and advocate condom use. He recognized the need to educate people about HIV and practicing safe sex.

Juanita's opinions reflected religious teachings and the prevailing climate of opinion in the barrio, but we have no evidence concerning how she might relate to issues surrounding HIV in private, among her own friends and family. In observations over the past decade, we have documented many occasions where she did not follow the religious rules she espoused. In these cases, Juanita assisted and supported her kin as much as she could. However, in the case of HIV, the vehemence of her condemnation and that of others associated with the Pentecostal Church stood in the way of community mobilization for prevention, if not in the way of individual care for people with HIV.

A second perspective on HIV prevention began to emerge in Yabucoa between 1989 and 1991. A small group of college educated people began to shift from categorical rejection of stigmatized groups to an understanding of the need for preventive measures. Some women recognized the need to develop grass roots approaches to prevention. In spite of continued discussions over three visits, no community groups emerged. Ida Susser talked most extensively with Dolores, a college-educated woman born in Yabucoa, with four teenage children. They discussed the necessity for women to work on prevention for themselves and Ida asked Dolores to gather a few women to meet as a group so that they might begin to raise community prevention issues. Although Dolores appeared concerned, no group ever emerged and it was not clear that such an approach could be effective at that point.

In 1991, Dolores' husband, Carlos, a high school teacher who was also a union leader and a local political figure was told that sixteen high school students in Yabucoa were infected with HIV. Up to this point, Carlos had not focussed on HIV as a community issue. He had, from the beginning, adopted a less condemnatory stance toward HIV than that espoused by the Pentecostal Church. He was a member of the Catholic Church with a belief in egalitarian reforms. He was shocked by the report of the 16 students with HIV and galvanized into action. Within a week he had pulled together a small group of community members to discuss HIV prevention with us. We agreed to help. After discussion with Dolores and Carlos, we invited two community organizers from San Juan active in HIV work to talk with the group.

At the meeting, only three husband/wife couples, all with teenage children, were present. The discussion turned immediately to how to address the problem of educating youth in the community about HIV. The unspoken premise of the discussion was that only teenagers were at risk; that stable couples should not be a focus of concern or education; that the way to reach community members was through concern over their children. Many interventions, such as a broad-based community event, the showing of videos and the distribution of questionnaires about knowledge of HIV in the community were discussed. Both men and women in the group demonstrated a high level of energy and commitment to the issues. However, in this setting at least, only high school students were viewed as possibly engaging in risky behaviors.

Observation of the formation of this group might be fruitfully compared to an earlier analysis of gender and political mobilization in Yabucoa (Susser 1985, 1991). In 1982, we conducted research concerning the emergence of the grassroots environmental movement opposed to pollution caused by a Union Carbide plant in Yabucoa. The dynamics of the movement were as follows: Women documented the possible health effects of pollution noting skin rashes among infants who crawled on dusty floors and increased asthma attacks in children. In response to the women's concern, men in the barrio, and later at the plant, organized to protest the pollution. Although women were active in generating and supporting the movement, the men took the public leadership roles in these activities[7] for over seven years. This should not be taken to indicate women did nothing. One woman in particular, the wife of the leader of the movement, exercised strong influence not only over the women involved with the movement but also the young men. But, she did this from her kitchen. Only in the last few years, with the departure of Union Carbide and waning interest in the protest, has a woman led what is left of this movement.

The activities initiated around HIV prevention may be following a similar path with respect to gender roles. While some people were aware of the problems and concerned with prevention since 1989, it was only in 1991, when a man who was a leading political activist espoused the cause that concrete actions were taken. When a group did emerge it was clearly based on cooperation between men and women in a similar way to the Union Carbide protest. The men were moving toward taking public roles and the women's discussion indicated they were preparing a supportive "home bound" participation. In neither instance, did women and men form opposing or alternative groups in recognition of gender inequality. On the contrary, in both instances the health issue was seen as a threat to the community and to families. It was perceived to be an issue which should be confronted by men and women working together, with men taking the public leadership roles.

The formation of this sort of group, consisting of married couples, specifically to lead a community grass roots effort in HIV prevention may, in fact, have limited the topics which could be discussed. The concentration on the threat of infection to teenagers was safe and embarrassed no one. Not only labor migration but other aspects of life in the barrio created the context for a risk of HIV infection among married as well as single adults. However, the negotiation of safe sex among couples, adult drug use or the question of sex between men were never raised by this initial group. It remains to be seen whether other grass roots groups may approach HIV prevention from a broader perspective.

In order to explain the process of organization found in the protest against Union Carbide and mirrored again in the formation of a group to prevent HIV infection, two aspects of life in Yabucoa will be explored. The first concerns the centrality of women in addressing household health. The second involves the differential socialization of men and women and its implications for group mobilization. To restate these questions slightly differently: the first question concerns why women were the first to understand and worry about the general risk of HIV infection in the community. The second question explains why women alone could not organize a group to discuss the problems. They were not able to publicly inform residents of realistic household concerns in opposition to general attitudes of categorically stigmatizing risk groups.

On the basis of previous research conducted with the environmental movement and our observation of changing women's roles over the decade of the 1980s and their emergence to leadership positions in the environmental movement (Susser 1991), we had come to the conclusion that women would be central to organizing

HIV prevention in Yabucoa. We mistakenly believed that a group formed by women would emerge on the basis of their understanding of the importance of HIV infection and the need to empower women to negotiate for safe sex.

It was only after three years of intermittent discussion and observation that we finally came to realize that effective organization in Yabucoa involves both men and women. Despite dramatic changes in the economic position of young women, their control over reproduction and their access to education, effective mobilization at the grass roots followed the same gender patterns as the mobilization efforts of the late 1970's and early 1980's. Ida Susser realized that her own "feminist" analysis of political protest and the needs for gender negotiation in HIV prevention was perhaps misleading or too narrow. In Yabucoa, at the present time, organization is founded on cooperation between men and women, based on a history of gender differentials in socialization, spatial mobility and access to networks. For the same reasons, however, it is still limited to a discussion of "others," i.e. teenagers, rather than the more problematic negotiations between men and women themselves.

Women's Concern With Health

Women both act and see themselves as the guardians of the family and the repositories of knowledge about health in the barrio. This potentially puts them on the front line in the battle against HIV infection and makes women's knowledge and perceptions key to the development of interventions. In 1982 and 1983, we interviewed people in 94 households about the health of other household members. When we asked questions about children's health, the men gave general answers or suggested we ask the women for detailed histories. Mothers, grandmothers and the sisters of mothers provided us with chronologies of childhood asthma problems, ear infections and skin infections. They remembered the dates the illnesses had occurred and on occasion, brought the medicine to show us what had been prescribed. Women were also well-informed about preventive health care, well-balanced diets and the health problems caused by unclean water and other sanitation inadequacies.

Working in the barrios in 1987, we found both men and women were aware of HIV infection in the community and one group did not appear more or less well-informed than the other. Women however, appeared more willing to state their fear of AIDS and may have been more judgmental of sexual behavior than men. By 1990, each adult woman we spoke to, several of whom had not finished high school and seldom left the barrio, knew the modes of transmission for HIV and knew that it could not be transmitted through casual contact. However, HIV prevention requires not only knowledge about health and transmission but the ability to discuss sexual activities with partners and others. We are not sure that women are able to take measures in this direction at this time, nor are they likely to be able to openly discuss intimate sexual matters. Though we might bring these matters up with the women, these issues were never raised by women in our conversations about health.

Socialization of Men and Women

In spite of their knowledge and concern for health and their fundamental role in maintaining family and community, entrenched gender roles in Yabucoa have so far limited women's abilities to lead grass roots initiatives for HIV prevention. In Yabucoa, women's social lives were distinctly different from men's. The differences in mobility for men compared to women was one of the greatest contrasts, which then defined also the locus of conversation and meeting places. If not employed, women were nearly always in the house, and that was where they were expected to be. Men, whether working or not, were seldom home and that was the way it was expected to be.

Division of tasks and socialization started at an early age. Most eight year old girls were already competent dishwashers, moppers and sweepers. The boys learned none of these chores and were left to run free in the yard or to wander the relatively safe streets of the barrio. By the age of thirteen or fourteen, boys seemed to disappear from the home environment and only appeared for meals and to sleep. Teenage girls stayed closer to home, under the tight jurisdiction of their parents. Young unmarried women left the house for work and training and were not in the kitchens as consistently as their mothers had been. However, even their freedom was curtailed in comparison to their brothers.

The tendencies for men to congregate away from home and women to stay near the kitchen determined their style of participation in grass roots organization. Men drove daily around the barrios, into nearby towns or as far as San Juan absorbing information, affirming long standing political connections and developing new contacts. However, while women stayed home, they consolidated kin networks and analyzed issues with neighbors and friends. The strengths and limitations of each of these roles are reflected in the consistent patterns found in the Union Carbide protest and the efforts to mobilize for prevention of HIV infection. Women might raise health issues in discussions with kin and friends but they still rely on men to pull community members together. Though the situation is changing, there are still two distinct arenas of activity in the barrios of Yabucoa, in a sense two separate fields of activity defined by gender.

Changing Patterns in Women's Roles

While the two- tiered division of social life in the barrio remains intact, women have been struggling in the household and the work place to renegotiate their gender roles. Young women are taking the initiative in limiting family size (two children instead of six is now both the ideal and the reality for many families); they are also seeking birth control sooner. In the barrios, women born in the 1950's almost universally use sterilization for contraception. Although sterilization is still the most prevalent form of family planning, some younger women consider birth control pills a viable option. However, even in 1991, no woman we spoke to was willing to consider using a diaphragm or discussing condoms with a male partner.[8]

There are additional small signs of change. Men appear to be assisting more in household tasks such as washing dishes, although this still remains occasional. New chemical processing plants and fast food chains in nearby towns hire both young men and women, and some women have been appointed to supervisory positions. Some women drive themselves to visit relatives and friends and young teenage girls grasp as much freedom as they can wrest from their households. Under these conditions, it is not surprising that women have also emerged as visible public leaders in community protest.

In the Union Carbide protest, negotiations and confrontations between the corporation and the community progressed through several phases. The roles played by women changed even while they retained responsibility for their households. Their initial concern precipitated the broad and long lasting movement led initially by men and later by the women themselves. During the period of the Carbide protest, the situation of the company, the workers and community residents were all changing, but simultaneously job opportunities for women and their ability to negotiate housework and reproductive decisions in their households were also changing. The changes in women's attitudes and behaviors in Yabucoa are reflected to some degree in the protest movement. If the general direction of these changes are reinforced, women might yet serve the community well in containing the HIV epidemic. If women can face up explicitly to limitations still imposed by their roles they might find the means to clear the way for negotiations for safer sex with their men and provide the impetus for a genuine and effective community based movement.

Conclusion: Prospects for an Effective Response

In this chapter, we have been concerned with the changing perceptions of HIV infection over time and among different groups and the way in which a response to the epidemic can be launched in rural Puerto Rico. While there are a number of factors which make grassroots organization difficult, there are also elements which can be enlisted in stemming the epidemic. The early movement around environmental contamination directed against Union Carbide is an example of the ability of the people of Yabucoa organizing to protect themselves from a perceived threat. But this movement illustrates one of the ways in which politics in Puerto Rico is conducted. Groups such as the one active in the Yabucoa area and centered in Barrio Ingenio, are active on the island at most periods. At the time we began work in Yabucoa and Barrio Ingenio, there were at least a dozen active and militant environmental groups on the island. Just prior to the period we began work on the island, Puerto Rico experienced the Rescate de Tierras (Rescuing the Land) movements in which landless rural people seized land en masse.[9] During the mid-1980's. there was a resurgence of fundamentalist Christianity which culminated for one sect in the foundation of Ciudad Christiana (the Christian City) not far from Yabucoa. A group of people from different municipalities coalesced to form a village based movement—for which they founded a village.[10] In addition to being a common feature of the Puerto Rican political landscape, political groups and their actions attract and hold the interest of the Puerto Rican populace in general. They are a standard feature of the six o'clock news. The potential significance of such groups for education around HIV infection is clear. The general mode of organizing at the grassroots level is well established; it is one of the ways of "getting things done" when political leaders fail to take the lead. In fact, it is one way that local people use to pressure their elected officials into action. The question which remains is whether or not such groups can be mobilized in effective interventions to prevent the spread of HIV and, hopefully, as a base of support for people with AIDS.

We believe there is the possibility for organizing at the grassroots level in Puerto Rico; but, we might note that the effectiveness of this response depends, in part, on the willingness of the United States to do something about the epidemic on the mainland. It will do little good if the people of Yabucoa mobilize while the government of the United States continues to proceed as though the epidemic were not worthy of a serious response.[11]

The epidemic came to Puerto Rico through the return of those who had been driven by the necessity to find work in the United States. Bonds of kinship and changing employment opportunities brought many back. The epidemic found a foothold in Puerto Rico, and it has spread faster and more extensively on the island than on the mainland. Even in the face of this rapid spread, resources that might slow transmission have been inadequate.

One theme of this chapter has been that specific socio-economic factors fostered the spread of the virus into the Puerto Rican countryside. While the main source of infection for men is intravenous drug use (Colon et al. 1991), the main source of infection for women is heterosexual sex. As noted above, this accounts for nearly one half of the cases of HIV infection among women.

A second theme of this chapter has been gender hierarchy and the way in which this bears on the development of interventions. It is our contention that containment of heterosexual transmission must take changing gender roles and households shaped by migration into account. "Education," in its conventional sense, is likely to achieve rather little. Men and women will not lightly agree to remain celibate, nor is it likely they will achieve lifetime mutual monogamy. Thus far, men have not typically been persuaded to adopt consistent use of condoms. Advice to restrict sex to known safe partners, difficult to follow everywhere, is unreal in a society in which geographic separation between partners is a norm for long periods: Neither partner can know [and perhaps does not want to know] of the sexual activities of the other during these separations. People want children, but the condom is a contraceptive device; there is, thus, a conflict between serious life goals and prevention (Stein 1990; Mays and Cochran 1988). These factors all bear upon how effective interventions may be and they require that women be empowered to aid in dealing with them.

Neither the social effects of migration nor a gender inequality will be easily dealt with at the community level. Nevertheless, it is at the local level by local people that the appropriate responses must be made (La Cancella 1989).

The communities of Puerto Rico possess several potential counter forces to the negative factors noted above: women and men are challenging and renegotiating established inequality in gender—the definition of gender roles is in flux; there is a history of effective grassroots mobilization around health issues, and other political issues as well; both in the barrios in which we have worked, and others on the island, positions of community leadership have been assumed by women as well as men. On the basis of these fundamental elements of community life and conditional on the committed support of financial and educational resources from San Juan and the United States Government, it is clear that effective prevention can be instituted among the majority of people in Puerto Rico who live outside the central cities.

At present resources and information are not flowing to rural areas in appropriate ways. Television messages alone lead to alienation and the stigmatization of groups; and, we are doubtful about the effectiveness of such messages, particularly in their current bland and uninformative form. With outside support, grassroots organizing could build on community strengths to empower men and women to protect themselves in a fluid social environment.

Gender roles are changing in a slow process we have documented over the past decade. Women have gone out to work, extended their education, changed their use of birth control and limited the size of their families. In order to prevent the spread of HIV infection, further challenges to established gender patterns need to be initiated. Further research is also required to evaluate whether groups in which men and women work together in HIV prevention are, in fact, able to address intimate issues which bear simultaneously on AIDS prevention and sexual equality.

The possibilities for change clearly do exist and, given resources and support, residents of Yabucoa will make the changes necessary to protect themselves and their children, as they have adapted their lives and households to other national and international forces.

Notes

1.   For a somewhat different perspective—but one which nevertheless agrees on all the essential features concerning the economic development of Puerto Rico and the place of migration see Raymond Carr's *Puerto Rico: A Colonial Experiment* (1984).

2.   The relationship of migration to states of ill health is well established (see: Susser, Watson, Hopper 1986); and its relationship to AIDS transmission, in general, is fairly clear (Micklin and Sly 1988; Kreniske 1988; and Kreniske this volume)

3.   In interviewing men at the local ballpark in the barrio as well as in the bodegas (small stores which also serve as bars and gathering places for men) it was interesting the degree to which men lacked information about life in the United States. In fact, even when told by recent returnees, many simply would not believe that the conditions described could

exist in the United States. They also could not believe that they would be subject to discrimination in the United States—even when returned migrants with many years experience in the United States gave catalogues of specific incidents. Lack of knowledge about the conditions encountered in the migration is not necessarily due to lack of information but rather, in at least some cases, to disbelief.

4.   One young man interviewed said he did everything he could to keep his addiction secret because if anyone found out he would be shut out of neighborhood society.

5.   The need for keeping this aspect of Barrio life in perspective is highlighted by recent remarks of the vice president of the Board of Education of New York City, Dr. Irene Impellizzeri. Specifically, Dr. Impellizzeri is quoted in the Spanish language press as having said that unlike Irish, Italian, Jewish and Asian immigrants the new Hispanic immigrants lack a high sense of morality (Rudy Garcia *Noticias del Mundo* 6/17/92). Such an assertion is patently absurd and reveals a deep ignorance of the character of life among Latino immigrants in New York. For the most part, this is a poor population and is subject to the pressures that poor populations of whatever origin have suffered. Their responses have been similar. In particular, however, many segments of this population have demonstrated great energy and enterprise in constructing new lives under difficult conditions.

6.   All names used in this chapter are pseudonyms.

7.   The way in which men took the public lead and the way in which they selected a leader is suggestive of *caudillismo*—to the institutionalized following of a charismatic leader. Leadership is on the basis of admirable personal qualities and, in politics, may have little to do with actual policies.

8.   In discussions with John Kreniske, the men were equally ill at ease in discussing condoms. They would make jokes or change the subject in an attempt to conceal discomfort. Some attitudes may not have changed over time. Similar discomfort was described by Sidney Mintz over thirty years ago (1960).

9.   The Dominican Republic and other islands in the Caribbean experienced similar movements at about the same time. In Puerto Rico, the most famous of these was Villa Sin Miedo (Town Without Fear). Of all of the groups engaged in seizures, this group had the most self conscious ideology and engaged in frequent confrontations with the police. In 1979, they were burned out of the site they occupied and wandered from area to area until they were given land by the Catholic Church on the side of El Yunque, the site of Puerto Rico's rain forest, in the late 1980s.

10.   The village purchased land about ten miles from Yabucoa. Unfortunately the land, and the stream that ran through the village, were contaminated by mercury possibly from local industries. Two children died and a number of people were hospitalized. Just a few years after being established Ciudad Christiana had to be abandoned and its population was dispersed around the island.

11.   We know how much and for what monies are being spent by the American Federal government. But, it remains true that the United States has no national, effective anti-AIDS program and that even its most recent efforts have been seriously criticized.

5

AIDS Prevention, Treatment, and Care in Cuba

Sarah Santana

Introduction

Among Caribbean countries, Cuba's response to the epidemic of human immune deficiency virus (HIV) infection merits attention because it is a comprehensive effort in a poor country that includes early, integrated, nationwide action. The epidemiologic characteristics of HIV antibody positive persons in Cuba are somewhat different from those in other Caribbean countries. Cuba's experience in screening large numbers of healthy individuals leading to long-term follow-up of asymptomatic HIV antibody positive persons could broaden the knowledge of the natural history of the disease. Cuba is the only country admitting into sanatoria both ill and healthy HIV antibody positive individuals. The Cuban program includes five components integrating preventive and treatment approaches:

1. Protection of the blood supply.
2. Widespread screening to identify seropositive individuals.
3. Educational programs for the general population, for specific high risk groups and for seropositive individuals, their friends and families.
4. Treatment of seropositive persons through a "sanatorial regimen" that includes temporary, partial isolation. This institutionalization has the double purpose of providing the seropositive persons with the best quality of medical care and living conditions possible and interrupting transmission by preventive education and limiting his or her access to new, uninfected sexual contacts.
5. Clinical research.

Background to Cuban AIDS Policy

The Cuban program and the Cuban HIV epidemic must be studied within the socioeconomic, political, cultural and ethical context of Cuban society. Cuba is quite different from other socialist countries in culture and history and from other Latin American and Caribbean countries in its political, ideological and economic systems. The epidemiology of HIV, the factors affecting who becomes infected, as well as the measures undertaken to control the epidemic are very much determined by this context.

Cuba is the largest island in the Caribbean with an area of ll0,000 square kilometers and a population of approximately 10.5 million, 67% of whom are 15-64 years old, with an excess of males in most age categories. The male/female ratio ranges from 1.01 to 1.04 for all age groups except for those 50-64 who show a ratio of .992 (MINSAP 1990a).

A revolution overthrew dictator Fulgencio Batista in 1959. In l961 the government officially declared Cuba a socialist state. Education and health services are free, housing and food costs represent a very small percentage of household income (Benjamin 1984). Malnutrition, acute poverty and many infectious diseases have been eradicated (Benjamin 1984; Muniz et al. 1984).

Some social ills affecting the patterns of HIV transmission in other countries, like IV drug abuse, are non-existent. Others, like prostitution are minimal. Individual prostitutes work mostly in Havana and nearby tourist centers and have been estimated to number in the hundreds (Manuel 1987). Because the prostitution trade is not in money, but mostly in consumer goods available only with foreign currency, and because pre- and extra- marital heterosexual relations are commonly accepted among the Cuban population, clients of prostitutes are mostly foreigners (Faas 1991; Manuel 1987). Although occasional gay prostitutes exist, gay prostitution is not widespread. All these conditions affect the pattern of transmission of HIV, which is very different from that observed in countries where prostitution and IV drug abuse are common. Up to October, l990, the most common risk factor for HIV in Cuba was having had sexual relations with a foreigner or with someone who had sexual contact with a foreigner (Terry et al. 1989).

Homosexuality is not illegal, but there is a strong cultural bias against it. During the last 20 years the state has not actively persecuted homosexuals, although they are still victims of unofficial social discrimination. There are no gay bars or baths where casual sexual activity occurs. Places where people meet both heterosexual and homosexual casual partners exist, but they are rare, especially outside the largest cities.

Travel into and out of Cuba has been routinely controlled and monitored since 1960. The state can identify most Cuban residents who have traveled abroad Terry and Rodriguez, personal communication). Until recently, Cuba had large numbers of citizens studying or working abroad with civilian delegations in over 30 countries and troops mostly in African countries (Grundy 1980; MINSAP 1989; Feinsilver

1989). Serving abroad is looked upon as an honor, it is those the society wants to reward and those committed to its goals and ideology who travel and have contact with foreigners. Therefore, the individuals at highest risk of infection are not minorities or "underclasses" of the society as in many other countries.

Cuba has a single, unified health system (Santana 1990) locally administered, with professional oversight at the national level. It has a widespread network of primary health care centers and family physicians, secondary and tertiary care hospitals and research institutes. The health profile of the population is more like that of a developed country than a developing one, with low infant mortality, low fertility, low rates of infectious diseases and high cancer and cardiovascular disease rates. Over 95% of pregnant women receive prenatal care and 98-99% of newborns are delivered in hospitals. There is very high utilization of primary and secondary health care services (Santana 1990; Massabot and Tejeiro 1987).

The health care system is based on certain operational principles, unchanged since 1961 (MINSAP 1969; MINSAP 1970):

1. Health is the responsibility of the state and the right of the people.
2. Care must be comprehensive, integrating curative and preventive services.
3. Care must be free and accessible to all.
4. Social services, health care and the socioeconomic development of the population are to be coordinated.
5. Popular participation in the health system is fundamental.

Although the health delivery organization has changed throughout these last 30 years, it has been a rational development which has built upon the solid bases of these principles (Santana 1987). The system relies on a network of community-based health teams (family physician and nurse) backed by extensive secondary and tertiary care institutions (Santana 1987; Gilpin 1989).

The population is well organized in each community. Over 85% of residents belong to one or several mass organizations such as block associations, the Federation of Cuban Women, associations of small peasants, students associations, etc. (Massabot and Tejeiro 1987; Reguera and Benitez 1979). These groups traditionally work in health activities such as health education and follow-up of the chronically ill. This and the large proportion of the population reached by the health system make it possible to have mass health-oriented campaigns with very high participation and acceptance by the population. These campaigns include immunizations, blood donations, and cervical cancer and HIV screening (Massabot and Tejeiro 1987; Reguera and Benitez 1979; Torres et al. 1987).

The emphasis in Cuban education at all levels is on self-sacrifice, the common good and the subordination of the desires of the individual to the needs of the nation (Wald 1976). Most people actually behave this way, either out of conviction or out of peer pressure. Part of this collective mentality is the expectation that the government will take care of all health needs, individually and collectively, and protect society from any public health threat. These factors seem to influence the apparent lack of resistance to admission to the sanatoria and the seeming societal consensus about this measure.

The HIV Control Program in Cuba

The National Commission for Control of AIDS was established in 1983. Its objectives were to ascertain the level of HIV infection in the Cuban population, and develop a program for the diagnosis, management and epidemiologic control of the disease.

Surveillance was instituted in 1983 in all hospitals. No cases were identified prior to the beginning of screening. The first AIDS case (not the first HIV antibody positive individual) was identified in 1986, presenting pre-mortem at the hospital and not through screening. In 1985 Cuban health authorities began planning, training personnel and purchasing equipment to carry out widespread HIV screening. By the end of 1985, all the elements were in place to begin the program.

Cuba's response to the HIV epidemic has been no different from its response to any other health crisis. Almost every health worker interviewed, at all levels of the health hierarchy, immediately mentions the dengue epidemic as an analogue to the HIV epidemic (Faas 1991). MINSAP has a very strong surveillance program with virtually complete coverage of the country and responds to rising numbers of cases of any disease immediately.

Thus, an increase in gastroenteritis, measles or meningitis in a municipality or province is immediately detected and measures taken. Even when there may not be much the health authorities can do, the population is informed that MINSAP knows and is doing everything possible to deal with the situation. This happens again and again, whether the disease is conjunctivitis, dengue, or HIV infection.

The legal bases for the HIV control program are originally set by the Cuban Constitution of 1976 which guarantees to the people free curative and preventive care, hygienic and occupational health protection and social security. It lists as one of the duties of the citizens full cooperation with whatever preventive public health measures are instituted by MINSAP as provided by law (articles 46-49 and 63, Chapter 6 of the Constitution) (Tabio 1985). In addition, it allows for the limitation by law of individual civil rights in order to preserve the peace, avoid public disturbances, encourage the common good, and "protect the existence and purposes of the socialist state and the Cuban people's decision to build socialism and communism" (article 61, Chapter 6 of the Constitution) (Tabio 1985). This is the equivalent of the U.S. and English law principle of balancing the interests of the state versus those of the individual when limiting citizens' civil rights (such as using the criterion of "clear and present danger" or that of "compelling state interest" when limiting first amendment rights).

Further, the bases for health-related measures are provided by Law Decree 52, approved by the Council of Ministers in 1982, the Public Health Law of 1983 passed by the Legislative Assembly (both in effect before the implementation of the HIV control program), and the 1989 Penal Code (articles 187-199, Title III, Chapter 5 of the Penal Code), in which violations to the Public Health are listed (spread of infections, adulteration of medicines, air and water contamination, drug trafficking, reporting of communicable diseases and others). Cuban law provides for a 50 pesos fine for unauthorized leave from the sanatoria, and imprisonment if a person *knowingly* infects another.

It is with this mind set that Cuban health officials speak of the "epidemiologic opportunity" to prevent the spread of HIV when it had not yet infected many persons. The Commission decided to first screen and protect the blood supply. Because the disease was sexually transmitted, all persons exposed to possible intimate contact with foreigners were screened, regardless of their sex or sexual preference. Prisoners were tested on the assumption that high promiscuity in the prisons could cause rapid spread of the disease if introduced in that population.

The costs of the preventive and treatment aspects of the HIV program have been very high for a poor country like Cuba. According to figures provided by MINSAP (Faas 1991; Terry, personal communication) approximately $3,000,0000 U.S. were spent during the first screening year (1986) on equipment, reagents and other necessities that had to be imported from capitalist countries and thus purchased with foreign exchange.

Since then Cuba has produced its own screening tests (ELISA and Western Blot) reducing its yearly foreign expenditures. As of 1990, the approximate cost of one day's stay in a sanatorium was 42 Cuban pesos (Santana, Faas and Wald 1991). This represents approximately 6.5 million pesos a year (and does not include screening or education, or the residents' salaries, which continue being paid). Cuba's health expenditures for 1989 were 1,015,600,000 pesos ($97 per person), approximately 12 percent of the national budget, and a 3.7 percent increase over the previous year. Although total HIV costs represent about one percent of the Cuban health budget, As of October, 1990, there had been no competition among other programs for these funds. HIV expenditures have been new additions to the budget— at official exchange rates the Cuban peso varies between .75 and 1.00 of one dollar (Santana, Faas and Wald 1991). The recent economic crisis in Cuba may very well change this situation in the future.

Epidemiology of HIV in Cuba

The rates of HIV infection in Cuba are quite low. As of August 15, 1991, the total cumulative number of identified seropositive individuals since 1986 was 650. This represents a cumulative seropositive prevalence of approximately .60 per 10,000 inhabitants (84 AIDS cases, of whom 51 (61%) had died, are included in these totals). Average annual incidence for HIV for the period 1986-1991 was .115 per 10,000 population. Annual incidence for AIDS cases by year of onset of symptoms in this period has fluctuated from a high of .019 per 10,000 in 1988 to a low of .011

per 10,000 in 1989 and 1990. (Santana, Faas and Wald 1991; Whaley 1991; Cabrera 1991; de la Osa 1991; Peña et al. 1990; MINSAP 1990). As a comparison, U.S. incidence of AIDS *cases* diagnosed in 1990 was 1.72 per 10,000, and over 179,000 cases have been reported in the period 1981-1990, of whom 63% have died (MMWR 1991). In Puerto Rico, a country with a population about 40% the size of Cuba's, the AIDS incidence for 1990 was 5.22 per 10,000 (MMWR 1991). The prevalence of HIV infection among blood donors in 1987 studies in the Caribbean were as follows: Cuba, .004%, the Dominican Republic, 1.62%, Jamaica, 0.23%. That year the U.S. had a prevalence among blood donors of 0.02 (WHO 1990b).

The screening prevalence in Cuba appeared to decrease steadily. It ranged from a low of 42.0 per 10,000 tests in 1990 to a high of 1.49 per 10,000 tests in 1986 (see table 2) (Santana, Faas and Wald 1991, Whaley 1991; Cabrera 1991; de la Osa 1991; Peña 1990; MINSAP 1990). Army recruits in the U.S. showed a prevalence of 13.1 to 14.8 per 10,000 persons screened for the entire period 1985-1987 (Burke et al. 1988; Bundage 1990).

Such steadily decreasing rates in a screening program are a common phenomenon, to be expected as screening culls the population of older infections, and as the screening universe is gradually enlarged to cover lower prevalence groups, even if among specific high risk groups prevalence does not decrease. However, in the period covering October 1, 1990 to August 15, 1991, these rates rose to .79 per 10,000 tests, just below the level of that in 1987 (Whaley 1991; Cabrera 1991; de la Osa 1991). The annual incidence of newly-detected seropositive persons has grown by small increments yearly, although Cuba has not experienced the exponential increase seen in other areas of the world, either in asymptomatic HIV infections or in AIDS cases.

HIV infection in Cuba began as a largely male heterosexual disease. However, the proportion of HIV seropositive persons who classify themselves as bisexual or homosexual has been steadily, although slightly, increasing every year probably as a result of the higher number of partners among homosexual HIV positive persons than among heterosexual ones. During 1986 and 1987 between 25-30% of the men classified themselves as bisexual or homosexual. By November, 1991, when the total number of HIV antibody-positive persons was 676 (482 were males), this proportion had increased to approximately 52% (Freudenberg 1990). Another element in the apparent increase of infection among gay or bisexual males may be the difficulty in having educational efforts reach individuals at risk due to the lack of organized gay groups, and /or the ignorance of the culture and mores of the gay community among MINSAP educators.

The male to female ratio, consequently, shows a slight increase in the proportion of women. In November, 1991 it was 2.48, in May, 1991 it was 2.52, it was 2.65 in October of 1988, 2.66 at the end of 1989 and 2.68 in October, 1990 (Santana, Faas and Wald 1991; de la Osa 1991). At this last date, it was 1.6 among heterosexuals, by November, 1991 it had decreased to 1.19. The most likely explanation for the initial excess of men among the heterosexual subgroup was probably the greater opportunity for exposure of the males, since it was mostly males who had travelled abroad. A differential transmission rate between men and women seems an unlikely explanation given the decrease of the male to female ratio as a higher proportion of new infections are domestically acquired. Also, there is evidence in the Cuban data that transmission from male to female may be more efficient than that from female to male. Only 5.6% of male contacts of seropositive women were found to be infected, whereas 12.1% of the female contacts of seropositive men tested positive (Terry 1989; Santana, Faas, Wald 1991). Another explanation for such a high initial male to female ratio among heterosexuals is that some men who are bisexual or homosexual may have deliberately misclassified themselves as heterosexual. This is possible, although gay residents of the sanatoria believe it is unlikely to any significant extent (Faas 1991, Santana, Faas and Wald 1991).

Infections among adolescents (15-19 year olds) are increasing. In January, 1990, the largest 5-year age category among the cumulative total of seropositives was the 20-24 age group, and persons 15-19 represented the 5th largest category. The mean age then was between 25 and 29 years old. By January, 1991, the mean age had decreased to below 24, and during the first six months of 1991, adolescents (who in 1988 were in sixth place among age groups identified as seropositive that year) represented the largest single age group among those newly diagnosed (Santana, Faas, Wald 1991; Ariyanayagam 1991). This could mean an increase in either the infection or detection rate among teenagers and may in part be a result of certain educational decisions made early in the program (see section on education below).

Because of the high percentage of women who receive early prenatal care, seropositive pregnancies are identified early and women can have therapeutic abortions. Out of a cumulative total of sixteen seropositive pregnancies by October, 1990, four had been carried to term, resulting in three pediatric cases. One of them a girl (now deceased) was born prior to the beginning of prenatal screening. Up to August, 1991, no additional pediatric HIV positive cases had been identified (Terry et al. 1989; Peña 1990; MINSAP 1990:34).

Again, as of October, 1990, nine seropositive individuals had been infected by blood or blood products. Of these, seven were domestic cases (two hemophiliacs), apparently infected prior to 1986; two were infected abroad, including an occupational case (Terry et al. 1989; Peña 1990; MINSAP 1990).

The most common route of HIV transmission in Cuba is sexual. As of October, 1990, when the total number of seropositives was 497, 475 (95.6%) were infected sexually. Ten individuals (2.1%) were under study and their source of infection had not been identified. In January, 1990, approximately 60% of those who were sexually infected, had been infected by sexual contact with a foreign person, either in Cuba or abroad (MINSAP 1990). Therefore, the remaining represent a first, second, third, and in some transmission chains even fifth generation of Cubans infected by Cubans in Cuba. It is this type of transmission that can be expected to increase and that is being seen mostly among women, adolescents and bisexual/ homosexual men (Ariyanayagam 1991).

Three general patterns are discernible among Cuban HIV seropositive persons, by screening group. The first pattern, occurring primarily in the eastern-most provinces, shows the majority of infections acquired abroad, and is primarily a heterosexual pattern. A second pattern is observed in the central provinces where infections acquired from other Cubans in Cuba predominate, with those acquired abroad in second place. The third pattern, observed in Havana City, does not show a predominance of any particular group (Peña 1990). These latter two patterns show a higher percentage of bisexual and homosexual infections, which follows from the higher number of contacts declared by homosexual or bisexual seropositive individuals when compared with heterosexual ones.

As of November, 1991, 98 individuals had been classified with AIDS (MINSAP 1990; MMWR 1987a:36), including 38 deaths. The most common conditions resulting in the immediate cause of death have been opportunistic infections (pneumocystis carinii pneumonia, candidiasis, histoplasmosis, cytomegalovirus, toxoplasmosis, criptoccocus, criptosporidium) and cerebral atrophy (one of these cases presented dementia as the first symptom). As of November, 1991, only two cases of Kaposi's Sarcoma had been observed (Peña 1990; MINSAP 1990; MMWR 1987b:36).

Among the 69 AIDS cases diagnosed up to January, 1990 the incubation period ranged from a minimum of five months to a maximum of twelve years, and survival after diagnosis has ranged from one month to over three years (the latter value attributable to patients still alive at the time). Based on 335 persons whose date of infection was known, a Kaplan-Meier survival analysis showed a 65% cumulative probability of having an incubation period of eleven years of more. This was true for both women and heterosexual males, but for bisexual and homosexual males the incubation period corresponding to the same 65% probability was significantly shorter, 6 years. The average survival after a diagnosis of AIDS (not just HIV seropositivity) was nineteen months, with an 80% probability of dying before 30 months. This held true for all AIDS patients, regardless of sex or sexual orientation.

Cuban investigators believe that a possible explanation for the difference in incubation periods, is the higher number of sex contacts declared by the bisexual and homosexual patients who thus may be subject to more repeated infectious challenges to their immune system than the heterosexual patients. Once AIDS develops, however, there seems to be no difference in survival (Peña 1990; MINSAP 1990; Martinez and Torres, personal communication).

According to the figures provided by the Cuban authorities, as of April, 1990, 122 HIV infections were directly attributed to travel to Africa, either because the person was infected there or was infected by someone who had travelled there. Over 350,000 Cubans have served in Angola in military or civilian capacities, and thousands more in other parts of Africa (Terry and Rodriguez 1988; Grundy et al. 1980; MINSAP 1988; Feinsilver 1989; Azicri 1988). As of December 31, 1988, among the 424,928 tests applied to internationalists, there were 95 seropositives, accounting for 35.4% of seropositives identified at the time, and representing a prevalence rate of 2.0 per 100,000, roughly 4 times that of the general population at the time (Terry et al. 1989). There does not seem to be evidence to support the fear that Cuba's foreign aid activities in Africa would produce an explosive HIV epidemic at home. The prevalence among Cuban internationalists at this time of highest rates was about 7 times *lower* than that among U.S. army recruits in the period 1985-1987 (Burke 1988; Bundage 1990). In the Cuban context, however, it has been an important source of infection. After 1988, Cubans returning from Angola were tested before they returned to Cuba so that their HIV status was known to them and to the health authorities before their arrival (Rodriguez 1988, personal communication).

Like everywhere else, in Cuba certain behaviors define groups at higher risk of HIV infection. As of October 1990, persons who had sexual relations with a foreigner or with someone who had sexual relations with a foreigner, were the single largest risk group. Prostitutes seem to be at higher risk for this same reason (the estimate by the staff of the sanatoria is that perhaps ten of the HIV positive women at that time were prostitutes) (Santana, Faas, Wald 1991). Two other groups show high prevalence, blood and blood products recipients and persons with a previously diagnosed sexually transmitted disease (syphilis and gonorrhea have been increasing, but it is unclear whether or not it is a reporting artifact; blood donations have been screened for Hepatitis B using an ELISA since 1988, with an estimated prevalence among blood donors in 1989 of 1.2% (Muzio and Garcia 1990). There are no other common behavioral risks such as use of intravenous drugs.

Because there have been no studies on the average number of partners of HIV negative persons during any time period, we cannot say that promiscuity is a risk factor in Cuba, although it stands to reason that it should be. The average number of contacts declared for tracing by seropositive persons in Cuba (time periods vary) are as follows: among male homosexuals, 9; among male heterosexual 3.4; among females, all heterosexual, 3.7 (Terry et al. 1989). Two factors may be artificially raising the average of the females and lowering that of heterosexual males. In the case of the females, the average includes the small number of women who probably were prostitutes, and who had a very high number of declared contacts, and in the case of the heterosexual males, all averages exclude contacts abroad.

In studies done among positive and negative female contacts of HIV positive males, the number of sexual contacts, trauma during intercourse and anal intercourse were all significantly associated with infection (Terry et al. 1989; Santana, Faas, Wald 1991).

Given the screening and surveillance in place since 1986, time from infection to diagnosis of HIV seropositivity has become shorter. All 109 HIV seropositive persons identified in 1990 were infected in 1989 or later. There is virtually no lag in reporting once a case or carrier is diagnosed, given the centralization of the program and the traditionally strong and uniform reporting system (Martinez and Torres 1990, personal communication).

Blood Supply

In 1983 the importation of blood and blood products from countries with reported AIDS cases was halted. Officials report that Cuba is now self-sufficient in its blood supply. Since May, 1986 all blood donations are screened (Rodriguez, personal communication).

There are approximately one half million blood donations in Cuba yearly, 80% of them from men, 50% of whom are between 20 and 40 years old (MINSAP 1990; Rodriguez, personal communication). Thus, at the beginning of the program, testing blood donations was a relatively quick way to reach a large sample of sexually active males, in addition to insuring the safety of the blood supply.

As of January, 1990 there have been seven domestic transfusion-associated cases, all infected prior to 1986. Of these, two are hemophiliacs. There are approximately 500 hemophiliacs in Cuba (MINSAP 1990). As of October, 1990 approximately 2,500,000 units of blood had been screened and 34 of them (0.136 per 10,000) had been found to be HIV positive (Terry et al. 1989).

Even though persons who have travelled abroad and other individuals at high risk of HIV infection are advised not to donate blood, there is no self-exclusion mechanism by which, upon donation, such individuals can identify themselves as high risk. This adds an additional measure of risk to the blood supply. Persons who suspect they may be HIV-infected but do not want to ask for a test explicitly may donate blood as a way of finding out their HIV antibody status. This happens even though the testing of blood donors is not anonymous. Seropositive donors enter the process of confirmatory tests, contact tracing and sanatorium admission following the same protocols as those identified through other screening methods.

Screening

Population Screened. By August 1991, 10,780,414 screening tests had been performed, identifying 650 seropositive persons (four seropositives to HIV2 virus). Thus, in order to identify one seropositive individual, 16,585 tests were done (Whaley 1991; Martinez and Torres 1990, personal communication).

Cuban epidemiologists estimate that a substantial number of tests are repetitions. Many persons have been tested more than once, some several times since 1986. About 2 1/2 million of these tests have been to blood donors (400,000 to 500,000 per year). There is a very high percentage of persons who donate every year, so that their blood has been tested yearly. People working in certain trades are re-screened periodically, sometimes at semi-annual intervals. Seronegative contacts of seropositive persons are tested multiple times. The approximate number of persons tested by early 1990 was estimated to be between 60-75% of the number of tests. This is between 78 and 92% of the population between fifteen and sixty-four (Martinez and Torres 1990, personal communication).

The screening program began by testing blood donors in 1986 and gradually expanded to cover other population groups. At the present time groups being screened are as follows— the first six groups are the same population groups sampled for anonymous screening by CDC in the U.S. in order to estimate seroprevalence (MMWR 1988:37; Dondero and Curran 1991):

1. blood donors
2. pregnant women
3. adults admitted to hospital
4. persons diagnosed with other sexually transmitted diseases
5. prisoners
6. army recruits
7. Cubans who have travelled abroad since 1975 or have frequent contact with foreigners, e.g., workers in tourism or foreign relations
8. sexual contacts of seropositive individuals
9. the adult population of specific municipalities where clusters have been discovered, where there is a high incidence of sexually transmitted diseases or where specific high risk conditions prevail, such as active tourist centers
10. foreign students attending school in Cuba
11. foreigners who live in Cuba for extended periods of time

These last two groups are not reported in this paper. Seropositive foreigners living or studying in Cuba are returned to their country. Screening is periodically repeated at least once yearly in continually exposed groups such as workers in the tourist industry, for example, hotel personnel and taxi drivers. Others are tested every time they return from a trip abroad. At the individual level seronegative sexual contacts of seropositive individuals are closely followed, counseled and re-tested every three months. Foreign tourists and diplomats entering Cuba are not screened (Terry and Rodriguez 1990, personal communication).

Consent. Persons screened because their blood was drawn for other types of procedures, such as during prenatal care, hospital admission, diagnosis and treatment of sexually transmitted diseases or blood donation are not asked for explicit consent to perform HIV antibody testing. In these cases the test is treated as routine. Those tested in workplace or neighborhood screening sessions consent implicitly by submitting to the test, since they know the test is being performed. During screening of the general adult population in specific municipalities and workplaces some persons absolutely refuse to be tested (for example, 130 in Old Havana and nearly 3000 in Sancti Spiritus in 1988). They are not forced to provide a blood sample, but they are counseled about safe behavior on the assumption that they may be seropositive (Sanchez 1988, personal communication). However, it is clear that pressure from peers, neighbors, co-workers and health officials is very strong, and many who would have preferred not to be tested have, nevertheless, agreed to it.

HIV seropositive pregnant women are counseled but not coerced to have a therapeutic abortion (Santana, Faas, Wald 1991). There is little if any stigma associated with elective abortions in Cuba. Even though the numbers and rate of abortions have decreased greatly in the last 10 years, the use of abortions as birth control was widespread in the 1960s and early 1970s and still is among the young (Alvarez and La Jonchere 1978; Hollerbach and Briquets 1983; Masabot 1986, personal communication).

Screening and Diagnostic Tests. Enzyme linked immunosorbent assays (ELISA) are used as screening tests. They are confirmed with two additional ELISA tests, then Western Blot and radio immunoprecipitation assays. They are administered and processed at the provincial level in 45 diagnostic centers (these are epidemiology and hygiene centers that are part of the health system and are not used or established solely for HIV testing).

A central, national reference laboratory is responsible for quality control. Cuba has developed its own ELISA and Western Blot test kits, periodically sending them abroad for evaluation and comparing them with eight foreign commercial kits. This on-going evaluation of tests is at times impaired by the lack of foreign exchange and the United States trade blockade of Cuba (Hollerbach and Briquets 1983).

The national laboratory reports a low false positive rate after the third ELISA. This seems to be borne out by reports in the United States (Burke 1988; Schwartz et al. 1988). The Cuban test kits show a sensitivity of 100%, and a specificity of 98.3%, 98.83% and 98.93% in Cuban and foreign trials that included sera from persons with other immunodeficiency syndromes (Machado 1988, personal communication; Fernandez 1990). Using the lowest specificity estimate, no more than 31 false positives would be expected after the third ELISA when screening 6,408,656 persons in a population with a prevalence of .611 persons per 10,000 *tested* (the estimate of the situation prevailing at the end of 1988). Since different ELISA's are used as second and third tests, with even higher specificity than the Cuban test, this would actually be an underestimate of false positives (Schwartz et al. 1988). Further testing of these persons with Western Blot and radio immunoprecipitation assays would eliminate all false positives. Because the Cuban HIV prevalence among those screened is so much smaller than that among U.S. army recruits the predictive value of a positive test is lower (92.7%) than that reported for the U.S. recruits (99.5%) (Burke 1988). Among subgroups of the Cuban population with higher prevalence such as travelers abroad or persons with STDs the predictive value would be higher.

As of 1989, the Cuban reference laboratory had not found a negative confirmatory diagnostic test when the three ELISAs were clearly positive. Negative or ambiguous Western Blots have been seen only among those with borderline ELISAs near the cut-off point. Persons with borderline positive results in Western Blot and other diagnostic tests are followed in the community under very strict confidentiality, providing them with intensive counseling and support until a definitive diagnosis is made, in some cases more than one year later. Cuban officials emphasize the extreme care they take in confirming beyond any doubt the seropositive status of a person, since the consequences are so serious. For some individuals the correct diagnosis has required tests for HIV2, simian immuno deficiency virus, and if HIV is suspected from their clinical illness, but they show no HIV antibodies, a virus isolate is done. Only two of these types of cases have been ultimately diagnosed as HIV infected and institutionalized. The rest had other diagnoses (Fernandez 1990).

Education

The educational component of the HIV prevention program addresses 3 different population groups: seropositive persons and their families and friends, the general public, and those in high risk professions (for example, the merchant marine, the military, civilians whose work takes them abroad, people in the tourist industry).

Accounts by health professionals and seropositive persons themselves describe as excellent the educational efforts directed at the residents and their families, which includes printed materials, films, videos, live talks and one to one sessions with the seropositive persons, their families and friends.

The AIDS/HIV preventive education for persons in high risk occupations has consisted of talks, printed materials and videos. The education of the general public has been large scale, although it may not have been maximally effective. Radio programs in the hundreds have been broadcast. As of September 1989, an estimated 6 to 7 million people have watched 33 TV programs about HIV. Newspaper and magazine articles about AIDS are published every week and literally millions of fliers, booklets and informational materials are distributed through workplaces and schools in many areas of the country (MINSAP 1989).

Cuban education has been factual and non-hysterical. The population knows HIV can affect anybody, not "just gay men" (the early impression, given by reports from the U.S.). Content is deemed congruent with Cuba's sexual culture, promoting behavioral change by emphasizing monogamy, "knowing" your partner and avoiding casual sex encounters. Condoms are mentioned but not emphasized and other "safer sex" methods are not considered culturally appropriate—the only sure prevention is "responsible" behavior. Free condom distribution is not advocated. MINSAP officials explain that if every non-monogamous sexually active person in Cuba, or any Third World country, used a condom in each sexual encounter, the expenditures for condom production, purchase and distribution would be unsustainable to the country.

The Cuban health system seems the ideal one to implement widespread and imaginative educational programs, tailored specifically to its population. MINSAP can command the full cooperation of all the media and, when necessary, of other state institutions like the Ministry of Education. The educational component of the Cuban program to control HIV infection has all the elements of a high quality and imaginative program but it took years for it to finally gel into a coordinated, effective whole. Expert sex educators were not initially included in the planning and implementation of the national HIV education program directed and executed by MINSAP (Terry and Rodriguez 1988).

Originally the exception rather than the rule, excellent popular TV programs have now been developed. Some address the transmission chains from individual to individual in understandable graphic terms, others show documentary footage about the sanatorium and interviews with HIV positive individuals, both gay and straight. Pieces in the written press, once dense with medical terminology, inaccessible or boring to many, have also improved. Since December, 1990, popular music, public art competitions and other activities aimed at young people have been used for AIDS education (Blanco 1991).

However, an educational program for high school students did not start until September 1988. As of October 1990, there had not been widespread study groups on the issue among the many mass organizations. Surveys and studies were conducted to determine educational preferences of the population (Faas 1991; MINSAP 1989), but the results were not immediately used to design programs. As a result, in spite of the high proportion of the population that has been exposed to information in the printed or electronic media, knowledge about the disease can be scant (Faas 1991, MINSAP 1989).

Because public education about HIV began later than all the other components of the program, it did not fully develop until later. This may have allowed infections to occur which could have been prevented, and may be a factor in the recently rising rates among adolescents. Increased emphasis has been placed on education in the last 2 years, including a new bureau of health education specifically for HIV work. The challenge to the educational effort now seems to be to reach the adolescents and the unorganized gay and bisexual men in the population.

Cuban health officials themselves emphasize that ultimately only education affecting behavior will prevent infection. At every turn the educational campaign on HIV waged by MINSAP insists on the importance of responsible individual behavior and the limited ability of the state in this situation to protect the population. But most people outside the sanatorium seem to feel that they are protected by the measures taken to partially isolate seropositive persons (Faas 1991; Santana, Faas, Wald 1991).

It is perhaps the lack of emphasis on individual responsibility in the prevention of disease among the Cuban population that sets the stage for the less than optimum performance of health education in general and specifically about AIDS. Contrary to the phenomena in the U.S. (Freudenberg 1990; Tesch 1986), in Cuba the population generally assumes that the state will take care of whatever problems arise. Collective solutions are offered and executed for all sorts of diseases, whether it is immunizations for measles or changes in the fat composition of milk. The health of the individual is a societal problem, and so, there is little precedent for placing the burden of prevention on individual behavior.

Treatment: The Sanatorial Regimen

Admission Process. Persons confirmed to be HIV antibody positive are interviewed by specialized physician and nurse epidemiologists in order to explain to them their condition and begin to plan their admission to a sanatorium. The individual's personal circumstances are taken into consideration, including family, employment, resources, housing, etc. The person's full salary continues to be paid, although they do not continue to work at their workplace. If they are unemployed, they are paid a stipend. Special attention is given to any domestic or economic problems, so that new housing is provided for the family should they need it, children may be placed in better or nearer schools, or their entry into a desired special school facilitated. A spouse's employment situation may be improved or changed as needed, and psychiatric and counseling services are provided to the family. Everything is free of charge.

The utmost care is taken in terms of confidentiality. Sexual contacts traced, whether ultimately seropositive or seronegative, are not informed who provided their name. Contact tracing personnel are chosen from among the most experienced staff in the program against sexually transmitted diseases. Many of them were trained prior to 1980 by personnel from the Centers for Disease Control in Atlanta, Georgia.

The individual decides whether or not (s)he wants to tell family, friends and co-workers of his/her HIV status. For persons who do not want to inform others, health officials provide elaborate and apparently effective alibis so that the person's absence from job and neighborhood is not attributed to his HIV status. For example, in some cases individuals appear to be transferred to another province to work, or to have gone abroad to study. These "covers" will not be good forever, but they seem to work for the time being.

I was pleasantly surprised at the extreme confidentiality and care taken with the privacy of HIV antibody seropositive persons, since neither the popular culture nor the manner of practice in Cuba places much importance on privacy (other patients are normally interviewed and examined in semi-private areas, conversations of the most intimate nature go on in waiting rooms and hallways, women have sonograms in group sessions and it is common to see people carrying on an intimate conversation from the sidewalk to a second story balcony—nobody seems to mind).

Treatment. The residents of the sanatoria have a special diet and exercise regimen. Pathogens are cultured periodically from different sites in each resident's body and the person is treated for all infections, even asymptomatic ones. Constant surveillance and a close patient-physician relationship lead to prompt treatment of opportunistic infections, following protocols accepted internationally. Pentamidine, AZT, acyclovir and interferon are used preventively and for cases classified as CDC group IV (Millan, personal communication).

According to reports from residents, the sanatorial regimen can both increase and alleviate their stress. Some residents say the stress of knowing they are HIV antibody positive is worse than anything else, and that they would have rather not known. Others say that knowing their HIV status and having everything in their lives taken care of, as well as being able to relate closely to other HIV positive people, has helped them relieve stress and cope with their illness (Faas 1991;

Santana, Faas, and Wald 1991). Even for these residents, however, the psychological distress produced by separation from family, friends and work has been considerable. The problem has been addressed by improved access to the world outside. The sanatoria are now temporary residences, and some newly diagnosed HIV positive persons are remaining at home, never becoming sanatorium residents (Whaley 1991; San Juan Star August, 1991).

Life in the Sanatoria. Cuban health officials changed and adapted the sanatorial system as it became clearer that there would be no effective curative agent or immunization available in the short run and that people would continue to be carriers for a long time. The goal now is the eventual re-introduction of still-infectious individuals to their communities after a period of separation rather than after a cure or after the population is protected by immunization.

Living conditions have become more comfortable. Residents of the sanatoria have moved to larger and better facilities since the inception of the program in 1986, now living in apartments housing 2-4 individuals per unit with what Cubans consider luxuries such as air conditioners and color TV. As of August, 1991, there were twelve sanatoria in as many provinces, so that seropositive persons can be closer to their homes while they are residents of the facility, and, once they return to their normal lives, they can have a specialized medical care unit within short distance.

The institution is staffed with health professionals specifically trained to work with HIV positive individuals. The residents receive periodic medical exams and have specific physicians assigned to each of them to assure rapport and continuity of care and management. They follow the same family physician system as the rest of the Cuban population, are under close epidemiologic surveillance and their special diet and exercise regimen is supervised. The facilities seem to have well developed recreation programs and the residents can continue their education in the sanatorium.

Some residents who have trades or professions that can be practiced individually, such as writers, artisans, physicians, nurses, office workers, accountants, economists, or computer programmers work in the facilities. Previously most residents were limited to institutional-type arts and crafts, and "make work" activities. The lack of productive work in the institution was a serious problem for people who live in a society that holds work and service to others as the highest honor and a person's most important function in life. This, however, is changing, and many residents now attend classes or have returned to live and/or work in their communities.

The patients are evaluated by the staff (psychologists, physicians, chaperons, nurses) according to their behavioral risk for infecting others, considering among other factors their family situation. Residents return to the community for visits, to attend parent-teacher conferences, for block association meetings. Family and friends can visit them as often as they wish, and they go home on the weekends, some accompanied by their families (parents, siblings, spouses, children), some chaperoned by medical students. By summer, 1991 less than half the residents had restrictions upon their sojourns outside the sanatorium (Cabrera 1991; Ariyanayagam 1991; San Juan Star August, 1991).

Spouses are admitted into the sanatorium if seropositive. If they have not seroconverted they continue to live at home and visit their mates whenever they choose. The couple is counseled, but they are not prevented from engaging in sexual relations. Gay couples are treated in the same way as heterosexual couples, whether they are both seropositive or not. The sanatorium is perhaps the one social, work and living setting in Cuba with the least discrimination against homosexual men, since they live together openly as couples, and share the exact same living conditions as other residents (Ariyanayagam 1991).

Debate on the pros and cons of the sanatoria is limited to residents, their families and staff at MINSAP, where the evolving consensus tends towards the return of most of them to the community. None of those interviewed outside these groups expressed disagreement with the policy, even though most Cubans tend to openly express their disagreement with many governmental policies as long as their criticism does not appear to be doubting the fundamentals of the Revolution or of socialism.

Discussion

AIDS seems to be a disease that, like an X-ray, highlights the flaws and weak points of every society. In many countries AIDS patients are homeless, have lost their jobs and salaries, have trouble paying for their health care, are shunned by family and friends and depend on "the kindness of strangers," private and religious organizations to survive. Most countries have not developed a comprehensive program to control HIV infection and provide care and treatment to persons with AIDS. Cuba, a poor, small country, has developed an HIV and AIDS program, treating this disease in the same manner it would any other.

When examined within Cuba's socioeconomic, political and cultural context, it becomes obvious, as Cuban health officials themselves state, that many aspects of the Cuban strategy to control the HIV epidemic, although logical and successful, are not exportable, especially to other Third World nations. Such a program requires a quick and flexible response from a single national health system with equal access to all, high utilization by the population and well organized communities. It requires acceptance by the population of mass screening; the ability of the health system to command the cooperation of other social institutions for the purposes of educating the public and to require that social welfare benefits be extended automatically and immediately to cover AIDS/HIV affected persons. It also requires the technological and economic capacity to manufacture and/or import the necessary equipment, techniques, and pharmaceuticals to screen the population and provide treatment for those infected.

It is not the purpose of this paper to discuss the ethical issues at play in the treatment of HIV carriers and AIDS patients in different countries. But the personal and societal costs of the "freedom" HIV carriers and AIDS patients have in other countries and of the type of care these persons receive in Cuba cannot be ignored. The Cuban program needs to be placed in the context of Cuban culture and society.

Cuban AIDS patients are provided with all their medical and material needs, whether or not their family and friends are supportive. The "sanatorial regimen" has helped isolate them from possible prejudice and discrimination. In exchange, they have been required to live for a time in an institution with limited and supervised contacts with the rest of the world. It is to the Cuban health system's credit that this is now changing and that eventually only those whose behavior is dangerous to others will be limited by compulsory residence in the sanatoria.

Each society has a different way of balancing individual versus collective rights when faced with phenomena it perceives as threatening to its health and integrity. Thus, the behavior allowed or required of a member of the community and the efforts expended to control the "threat" are different in each society. They depend on the perceived seriousness of the threat and the relative value placed on collective versus individual well-being. The behavior allowed or required of a member of a Mennonite congregation in Pennsylvania, or a resident of a small town in Holland is very different from what is allowed or required of an individual in New York or Amsterdam.

In Cuban society great sacrifices are demanded of the individual in the interest of their perception of a strong and healthy society not only in the case of AIDS patients, but in all situations. This attitude, although reenforced by the socialist state, has its roots in traditional Cuban history and culture. A phrase out of the Cuban national anthem (which dates from the middle of the nineteenth century) best sums up this attitude: "to die for the motherland means in fact, to live." In exchange for this sacrifice of privacy and individual freedom, the society provides the individual with a large measure of security, so that housing, health, jobs, education and a safe environment are guaranteed and do not depend on isolated individual actions, but on collective ones.

Institutionalization of HIV carriers is not an exportable model for many reasons. It is only possible early in the development of the epidemic, since it is not feasible (economically, socially or politically) to institutionalize large numbers of persons in this manner. Cuban HIV infected individuals, in contrast to those in other countries, have not been members of any minority group. They are not IV drug abusers, they are not an ethnic, racial or religious minority, they are not poorer or richer than the rest of the population, and only recently has a substantial proportion of them (about 1/3) belonged to the gay/bisexual minority. There has not been a danger of applying institutionalization differentially to any group.

The goals of the Cuban HIV program are to interrupt transmission by preventing new infections and to provide as good medical and supportive care as possible to those already infected in the hope that this will prolong their lives until an effective therapeutic agent is discovered. The Cubans truly feel that these persons deserve the full support of the society and have devoted large amounts of resources (especially for such a poor country) to these goals.

The Cuban program is constantly under modification. Technical advances in treatment and screening are adopted as soon as possible. Educational efforts are under constant expansion and new methods are incorporated yearly. The sanatoria themselves are under constant review and are now beginning to function, at least for many if not all HIV positive persons, as back-up ambulatory facilities to get care and support and not as permanent residences.

This has been the results of debates and struggles within MINSAP, and, as they themselves say, a "dialectic" process of adaptation of the intervention measures to the circumstances and the knowledge of the disease. This is typical and traditional behavior for the Cuban health care system (Santana 1987), and is reflected in the different wording, and tone, if not actual factual content of the declarations by various officials, patients and documents (Whaley 1991; Arayanagam 1991; San Juan Star August, 1991).

It remains still to be seen whether the Cuban program succeeds in lowering or stabilizing the rate of transmission in the country. Questions need to be asked in the specific Cuban context in order to evaluate the performance of the program. It is already evident that the screening program has been successful at identifying HIV seropositive persons before they develop AIDS symptoms. As of October 1990, only 9 of the 69 AIDS cases (and of the total 497 seropositive persons) had presented at a health facility with symptoms. During the year ending in November, 1991 only two persons presented at a health facility already suffering symptoms of AIDS. Others have been screened at hospital admission or other health service encounter and found to be seropositive, but their contact with the health care system was not HIV-related (Martinez and Torres, personal communication; Peres, personal communication).

Has the educational program succeeded in making HIV antibody *negative* persons aware of their own responsibility for protecting themselves and preventing further spread? Can Cuba's health education reach the groups whose incidence seems to be rising: the un-organized gay population and the difficult-to-convince adolescents? Does knowledge of HIV status encourage responsible sexual behavior, whether a person lives in a sanatorium or not? Will the persons that avoid testing for fear of institutionalization become a serious source of new infections in the population, or will they practice good prevention, even if evading the screening test? Has the sanatorial regimen been an important factor in preventing new infections, or has it been counterproductive by reenforcing unsafe sexual behavior among the population, who mistakenly rely on it as a measure of control? Has early identification, treatment, and optimal living conditions improved survival among HIV antibody positive individuals regardless of the stresses of institutionalization? Was the low prevalence observed in successive screenings a real effect of diminished transmission rates, or an artifact produced by the groups that are being regularly re-screened? What does the latest increase in detection rate mean?

The rationale expressed by Cuban health officials for the establishment of sanatoria was based in part on the belief that sexual behavioral change would take too long to achieve given the sexual mores, culture and the machismo of the Cuban population. In the meantime, the probabilities that seropositive persons would infect others had to be diminished. The belief that the sexual behavior of Cubans (males and females) cannot be changed was belied by condom sales. These increased by 38% during the first 5 months of 1988 when compared with the same period in 1987, and have continued to increase (Rodriguez, personal communication; Terry, personal communication). KAP surveys carried out since 1987 have shown that teenagers and young adults are much more accepting of condom usage than those over 21 years old (MINSAD 1989). All of fifteen university students interviewed at a coffee shop in Havana in 1989 and 1990 (ages sixteen to nineteen) carried condoms with them, made in Mexico or China, whether or not they actually used them. So, it seems there is enough receptivity in the population for education to effectively reduce high risk behavior.

No one in Cuba pretends that all transmission will be stopped by their evolving program. But they may have been able to reduce transmission enough to prevent an exponential increase in infections. Cubans think they may have gained enough time to allow for improved educational methods to affect transmission and for the possible development of immunizing and/or curative agents in the future. A thorough evaluation is still pending.

6

AIDS in Uganda:
The First Decade

George C. Bond
Joan Vincent

Introduction

This essay is written by two anthropologists who are not medical anthropologists.[1] It is our contention that the social science study of AIDS in Africa, requires the efforts of both anthropologists sensitive to public health, biomedical and non-western healing issues, and anthropologists who seek to analyze the AIDS epidemic as they would any other phenomenon occurring in the field. We further contend that an ethnographic approach, resting on the analysis of cultural, social, political, economic and religious dimensions of local, national, and regional entities, is required, not simply to relate the grapeshot AIDS data of the past decade but to further understanding and analysis of epidemics.

In this essay we focus attention on the recent history and politics of AIDS in Uganda. We begin by noting the primacy that has been accorded to AIDS in Uganda and proceed to trace social science involvement in AIDS research through three phases from 1982 to 1990. We then draw attention to what we call Hidden Uganda, a dimension of the AIDS epidemic in contemporary Uganda that has been completely unresearched and unstudied. This, since 1987, has been a context of civil war, military occupation, famine, and resettlement in northeastern Uganda. In very real terms, for anthropologists, this is the moving AIDS frontier. Concluding the essay we argue that, for anthropologists who are not medical anthropologists, medical conditions are a part only of the AIDS epidemic in Uganda.

Cases of AIDS were first recognized in the United States in 1981 and in Uganda in 1982. The Uganda findings were published in *Lancet* in 1985 under the heading "Slim disease: a new disease in Uganda and its association with HTLV-III

85

infection." This article's leading author, David Serwadda was a clinician attached to Mulago Hospital, the teaching hospital of Makerere University in Kampala.

After the initial clinical recognition of AIDS, epidemiologic research was initiated to discover transmissions patterns, risk factors, and the prevalence of HIV infection in Uganda (Serwadda et al. 1985; Sewankambo et al. 1987; Berkley et al. 1989; Hudson et al. 1988a; Carswell 1988). In collaboration with the World Health Organization, an AIDS Control Program (ACP) was set up in 1986 (Okware 1987). Between 1987 and 1988, most of its $14 million budget was spent on health education, the protection of health workers, serologic testing, and blood bank renovation. In 1988 Uganda's Ministry of Health called for more attention to patient care. In late 1990 a massive restructuring of AIDS research and governmental responsibility was undertaken with President Museveni himself at the helm.[2]

Anthropology and AIDS Through Three Phases

A series of switches took place between 1982 and August 1990 in the relation of medical to social science AIDS research. These epistemological developments were reflected in Ugandan AIDS research. Anthropological involvement passed through three phases:

1. Anthropologists as Handmaidens: The Biomedical Paradigm
2. Anthropologists as Social Workers: The Community Paradigm
3. Anthropologists as Social Analysts: The Critical Paradigm

We will review the roads taken and the roads not taken in each.

Anthropologists as Handmaidens:
The Biomedical Paradigm

In Uganda this phase lasted from 1982 to 1988. Its watchwords were "Love Carefully" and "Zero Grazing". Anthropologists were employed to carry out field inquiries among target populations which had been constructed for medical reasons. Studies of AIDS in Kenya and Zambia had shown an association of HIV infection with (a) increased numbers of sexual partners; (b) a history of sexually transmitted disease or genital ulcers; (c) the presence of an intact foreskin; and (d) a history of prostitution or sexual contact with a prostitute. Specific Ugandan studies contributed to this research (Hudson et al. 1988a; Berkley et al. 1989a; Berkley et al. 1989b; Carswell 1988).

Because of the ease of surveillance and policing on legalistic grounds, the "risk group" most often studied was "prostitutes." These were transmogrified in the Ugandan literature not to "sex workers" as elsewhere, but to "bar maids"! Serologic surveys carried out in Rakai district found that "barmaids" and truck drivers had exceptionally high seropositivity (67% and 32% respectively). This finding (Carswell 1988) was generalized to Uganda as a whole. Government efforts to control truckers' movements led to unpleasant incidents, even at the international level between the Kenyan and Ugandan governments. No anthropological study of truckers has been carried out in Uganda although Southall's (1980) essay on their transnational movement and black marketing activities provides a base which researchers into the spread and transmission of AIDS find highly provocative.

In 1988 a so called *national* serologic survey [of which more anon] showed rural seropositivity rates of 7-12% and urban rates of 8 to 30%. By 1990 it was observed:

> because of the high prevalence rates in the general population, knowing a patient's social history rarely helps in making a diagnosis of HIV infection. Old and young, rural and urban, married and single are all commonly infected. Similarly, members of all ethnic groups, religions, and professions are at risk (Goodgame 1990:383).

At this point, clinical attention began to shift to tuberculosis as a common manifestation of AIDS. This co-occurrence was first noted by Serwadda and his colleagues in their 1985 report on "Slim." Prior to the HIV epidemic, 16,000 new cases of tuberculosis had been reported annually. Between 1984 and 1987, the annual number of cases doubled (Eriki 1988). By 1989 pulmonary tuberculosis, tuberculous adenitis, pleural effusions, peritonitis, and pericarditis accounted for approximately 30% of medical admissions to Mulago Hospital. In 1990 it was projected (Goodgame 1990) that with 1 million Ugandan adults already HIV seropositive, there could be up to 50,000 new cases of HIV-induced active tuberculosis each year. This places Uganda among the highest incidence countries in the world.

Opportunistic infections in Ugandan patients with AIDS (Sewankambo, Mugerwa and Goodgame 1987) led to a questioning of the WHO clinical case definition for AIDS in Uganda (Widy-Wirski et al. 1988). Environmental exposure to crypto sporidia is considerable in Uganda which may explain why chronic diarrhea and wasting are the commonest manifestations of those presenting symptoms of AIDS. Gastrointestinal organisms such as salmonella, shigella, giardia and amoeba are endemic. There are also high rates of infections acerbated by HIV-induced immunosuppression: syphilis 5-30%, chronic hepatitis 15%. Clinical research was undertaken to determine the interaction of HIV infection with "the very common traditional tropical diseases found in Uganda: malaria, trypanosomiasis, filariasis, leprosy, and others" (Goodgame 1990:385).

Most of the anthropologists employed during this first phase were funded as members of biomedically oriented research teams by international and United States organizations such as WHO, AID, and the Rockefeller Foundation. They directed their inquiries almost wholly into commonplace heterosexual sexual behavior.[3] Perhaps because many of these anthropologists were young female pre-doctoral candidates, this tended in Uganda towards a representation of the plight of women at the mercy of promiscuous husbands and/or a creation of data on attitudes to condoms (Forster and Furley 1989). Because of the urgency of the research, the main modes of inquiry adopted—questionnaires and surveys—were hardly distinctive of fieldwork at its best.[4]

Several anthropologists became impatient with the medical profession's requests for more and yet more targeted research. They suggested its apparent ignorance of the existence of a great deal of relevant literature. The Australian anthropologist Larson pointed out forcefully:

> A rich source of data on contemporary sexual relations already exists in the corpus of published material based on decades of anthropologic fieldwork. *AIDS is too urgent a problem to be assessed by means of costly, time-consuming research that merely replicates other findings* (Larson 1989:716-717).

Larson's own review of this data was specifically designed to "explain the differences within [East and Central Africa] that can be useful in anticipating a worsening AIDS epidemic and in designing policies to thwart it" (1989:717). She focuses first on the development of cities and then the continued relevance of traditional (sic) cultural attitudes regarding marriage and sexuality.[5] Larson points out that focussing on unaccompanied women and prostitutes as the primary AIDS threat merely invokes longstanding prejudices about urban women and discourages people [presumably men] from thinking about whether it is their own behavior that puts them at risk.

Topics recognized as stereo typically anthropological elsewhere in Africa, such as "traditional healers" or "witchcraft" have received little attention in Uganda. This reflects, perhaps, the early *predominance* of the biomedical paradigm and its propagation in the southwest and south where the moving frontier of the AIDS epidemic was first encountered in Uganda. Maxine Ankrah, of Makerere University's Department of Social Work and Social Administration, drew attention to witchcraft beliefs among the fishermen of Rakai among whom AIDS was first diagnosed in 1983. She suggested that "belief and flight from witchcraft . . . conditioned the initial spread of the HIV infection in Africa"(1989:267). The significance of witchcraft in Uganda has been disputed (Obbo 1991; Lyons 1991). Ankrah herself provided a temporal perspective:

> the notion that witchcraft was responsible for the disease, a belief held so firmly in 1983, was largely denied in 1988. Yet, what the specific factors were that led to the abandonment of a socially significant explanation for illness, or whether indeed it still operates, was not examined. Therefore, what the contrasting viewpoints are, how strongly they are adhered to, the conditions and information leading to the adaptation of new belief systems, are questions that need to be answered. The danger is that low priority will be given to these questions (Ankrah 1989a:267).

The record of the past decade has, however, been one of "too much epidemiology, too little social science," Ankrah (1989a:267) argues.

Our research in Rakai in 1988 provides support for Ankrah's emphasis on the complexity of plural belief systems. The interplay among traditional healers, herbal medicine, "witch doctors" and the Catholic church was addressed in our unpublished report on Rakai (Bond and Vincent 1988a) and is touched upon in our published 1989/1991 article; it is the subject of a companion paper to this, "Medicine and Morality."

Further, we suggest that while Ugandan research remains focussed on the areas initially suffering most from HIV infection and AIDS (the south and southwest) religion, healing and morality may be accorded low priority as Ankrah suggests. But if it follows the moving frontier of AIDS to the newly pacified north and northeast, knowledge of "local knowledge" will become critical to AIDS intervention and control. In Soroti district in 1990, for example, an admixture of international pentecostalism with "traditional" Iteso beliefs in sorcery to account for illness and misfortune (Vincent 1971) existed alongside narrative accounts of soldiers' seductions and rapes to account for the rapid growth of AIDS among women.

Whether there is widespread "factual" awareness of AIDS throughout Uganda (Serwadda et al. 1990; Schopper 1990; Ankrah 1989a) was subjected to considerable survey inquiry in the 1980s. A mass media campaign was initiated in 1986 yet three KAP surveys (Serwadda et al. 1990; Konde-Lule and Berkley 1989; discussed by Schopper 1990:1266-1267) showed that fewer than half the Ugandans surveyed in April 1987 recognized the campaign slogans. In September 1987, 37% of 4000 adults interviewed believed that AIDS was transmitted by insect bites, and only 15% knew that AIDS was incurable.

Much of the readily available literature on AIDS in Uganda during this phase was intended for popular consumption and inclined to sensationalism and exoticism. Robert Caputo's article "Uganda: Land beyond Sorrow" which appeared in the *National Geographic Magazine* in 1987 and Ed Hooper's "AIDS in Uganda" which was published in the same year in *African Affairs* were typical. Both had considerable impact on biomedical research workers as well as on the reading public in Uganda. Most critical of all was their effect on Rakai district and particularly the Rakai village of Kasensero, which had come into the biomedical and public spotlight under the name of Goma. In September 1988 we found not simply fear and anxiety in Kasensero but resentment and anger. Residents in the fishing village given such notoriety by Caputo resented being treated as inmates of a human zoo by the medical teams of international AIDS agencies and journalists visiting Uganda's landmark "home of AIDS." We were shocked at the "common knowledge" of our driver about which villagers had AIDS and which did not (Bond and Vincent 1988a:34). Later the dehumanizing treatment that accompanied early medical intervention in Rakai bred short term resistance to serosurvey testing in several villages.

Grey literature that might have countered this sensationalism was produced by several of the new organs established by the Uganda Government for research into AIDS prevention and control. Yet its facts and figures entered medical science infrequently and sometimes incorrectly. This bio-medical accumulation of data was objectively targeted more towards the international AIDS community in the United States than towards Uganda and the rest of Africa.

We suggest that to a marked degree the development of a Third World "specialization" in AIDS knowledge, and, further, the development of "specialization" in Africa, has limited communication *within* the social sciences. The magnitude of this danger may be represented by an article by Richard Goodgame published in *The New England Journal of Medicine*. Immediately upon publication this was singled out for attention by the London-based Economist Intelligence Unit, one of the world's leading publishers of international economic analysis and forecasting. Goodgame, who was attached to the Gastroenterology section of Baylor's Department of Medicine in Texas, was funded by the Foreign Mission Board of the Southern Baptist Convention.[6]

The Economist's Intelligence Unit's Country Report for Uganda, No. 4 of 1990, bore the heading "A medical study of AIDS makes depressing reading."

As the AIDS epidemic continues to gather momentum, the implications of the disease remain, for the most part, a matter of speculation and uncertainty. The Ugandan government has made no secret of the widespread incidence of AIDS in the country and has initiated a vigorous campaign of public education under the "love carefully" slogan. However, everybody knows that the impact is worse than the level of reported cases (more the 15,000 by March 1990) might suggest and the authorities are understandably apprehensive about the damaging effects of unsubstantiated scare stories. In this context, the publication of an authoritative study of clinical and social aspects of AIDS in Uganda by Dr Richard Goodgame in *The New England Journal of Medicine* in August 1990 is clearly to be welcomed, even though it paints a bleak picture. According to this source, about 1 mn adults out of Uganda's 17 mn population are estimated to be HIV positive and AIDS is already the most common cause of admission and death among hospitalized adults in many parts of the country. High risk groups do exist, notably barmaids (67 per cent positive) and truck drivers (37 per cent), and most cases fall into the 20-40 age group. However, the general level of infection is already relatively high, at between 7-12 per cent in rural areas and 8-30 per cent in urban areas. Members of all ethnic, religious and professional groups are equally at risk (EIU 1990:15).

This was the received wisdom on AIDS in Uganda in 1990.

Anthropologists as Social Workers:
The Community Paradigm

"AIDS: The subject is human" (Ankrah 1989b:265) was Uganda's social science message in 1989. For the people of Uganda, "Love faithfully" began to replace the earlier yuppie slogan of "Zero grazing" and "Love carefully." Philly Bongoley Lutaya, a Ugandan recording artist, and an AIDS sufferer, replaced both with the less self—oriented message: "Love responsibly" (Hunter 1990:681). And, in the new phase of caring rather than curing, "The human face of AIDS" (Hunter

1990:681) tended to be that of the grandmother, the widow or the orphan rather than that of the AIDS patient. Just as the biomedical phase of research in Uganda from 1983 to 1988 had tended to seek out—and blame—the victim of the disease, so the second phase tended to focus on the social dislocation caused by his or her death.

Research shifted *from curing to caring* in response to mounting evidence of agrarian immiseration, vertical transmission of AIDS, the plight of widows, and, above all, a large population of orphans. Non-governmental organizations (NGOs) operated throughout much of the country by this time, some even working during the civil war period in the north and northeast where the government had not yet restored its authority.

In the well-worked southwest, overlapping and complementary research was conducted by an abundance of NGOs. A Protestant assessment of AIDS and the development needs of Rakai (Kaduru, Mwesigwe and Nambi 1990) marched alongside a similar (and yet dissimilar) report issuing from Catholic agencies. Our own first engagement with AIDS in Uganda was centered around the activities of Catholics and Muslims in Rakai; later we were able to conduct short spells of observation and inquiry in Jinja and Soroti.

A most important inquiry was conducted into what it cost a family to support a sick kinsman at Kitovu Hospital, a hospital in Masaka run by the Medical Missionaries of Mary. Two adults were required to look after each patient with AIDS with probably a third delivering food to the hospital now and then. So burdensome was this to the family of the patient that the hospital was now encouraging home-based care through counseling. This type of Phase 2 data was very different from the stereo typically "traditional" kind of social science research earlier conducted into AIDS. It also raised for the Ugandan government the question of whether allocation of international funds to the kinds of clinical research characteristic of the 1986-1988 paradigm was the soundest form of responsible political investment.

Ugandan resources for caring for orphans—historically and worldwide a *parochial* matter—was of primary concern. There are believed to be some 24,000 orphans in Rakai alone, 66% of whose parents' deaths occurred in or after 1986 (i.e. after the end of the civil war that brought President Musevini and his National Revolutionary Movement to power).

Definitions of "What is a child?" vary considerably in Ugandan research. In one study children were persons under 18 years of age (Muller and Abbas 1990). "What is an orphan?" also receives various answers. UNICEF's Elizabeth Prebble defines AIDS orphans as children under 15 whose mothers have died of HIV/AIDS (1990). Anthropology's newly awakened sensitivity to the politics of categorization as exclusion and inclusion and its role in legislating and policing society make these critical questions now for the present generation of Ugandans. A suggestion that many of the present orphan problems are not due to AIDS but to civil war (Muller and Abbas 1990:79), is clearly not supported by the Rakai evidence referred to earlier. The suggestion in itself reflects as much as anything else the infra structural lack of communication between NGOs and the controlled distribution of "grey literature" on the subject.

We suggest that Uganda's experience with AIDS orphans must be viewed not specifically as findings relating to Uganda, but findings related to a country which was among the first to report its AIDS problem to WHO and thus among the first to open its doors to international AIDS researchers. The Uganda AIDS experience must be read as a *precautionary* tale for nations that have not yet reached "Wave 3" (Erickson 1990) of the processual AIDS paradigm.

This is not the place to consider the implications of NGO activities for Ugandan sovereignty but we note that during this phase the government welcomed financial aid from international donors with only a few strings attached. Not until the third phase (to be discussed shortly) was an attempt made to centralize NGO activity and provide for closer communication among them. Pluralism fostered a predominantly decentralized perspective. This was also reflected in the changing policy formulations at the United Nations Development Program (UNDP) which began to urge a focus on "local communities" which became explicit in the 1990s.

Accounts of Ugandan community based organizations (CBOs) have been largely descriptive and incidental.[7] Such organizations include the AIDS Support Organization, TASO, formed in 1987 (Kalibala 1989) and the Uganda Women's Efforts to Save Orphans, UWESO (Larson 1989, Ankrah 1989a). They await analysis as, of course, do the funding agencies closely involved with Uganda's caring phase. These were UNICEF, Save the Children Fund (SCF), and the League of Red Cross and Red Crescent Societies.

This was a period in which the economic impact of AIDS was becoming more apparent. A Working Group on the Socioeconomic, Cultural and Legal Impact of AIDS was formed in Uganda in 1990. Studies of manpower in Uganda (Olowa-Freers 1990) appeared in the grey literature and Steve Barnett and Piers Blaikie carried out research in Rakai into "community coping mechanisms in circumstances of exceptional demographic change" between 1988 and 1989. Because of its "depressing" nature, their report did not see the light of day until July 1990 and then only in a truncated version. This Doomsday scenario generated by a study of an agricultural region coping *at the community level* with the mortality of the AIDS epidemic, demands that the government take a responsible position in planning for the needs of its citizens:

> Very high priority should be given to sensitizing senior administrators to the fact that AIDS has implications for their area of responsibility. The downstream effects of AIDS will affect employment policy, education and training, law and order, defense, the position of women in the family, property law, agricultural production, as well as the more obvious effects on health provision . . . A secondary objective should be to formulate internal policies to cope with the losses of staff through illness and death (Barnett and Blaikie 1990:xxii).

Anthropologists as Social Analysts:
The Critical Paradigm

By 1990 both medical and social scientists writing on AIDS in Uganda had adopted a more critical tone. In anthropology an anti-biomedical movement was in formation. The grey literature gave a clear impression in December 1990 that Uganda was bogged down in "AIDS complexities" compared with a country like Zambia where things seemed to be going much better (Bond and Vincent 1990a:2). We suggested, using Jonathan Mann's division of the AIDS pandemic into three "waves" (Erickson 1990) that each African government needed to assess its current policies and programs for intervention and control according to which of these waves it was riding. Advance planning might avoid, we suggested, many of the problems (particularly political problems) encountered in Uganda—the pioneer nation, as it were (Bond and Vincent 1990).

By 1990 Uganda had clearly moved through a wave of HIV infection and through the epidemic of the AIDS disease itself, to an epidemic of economic, social, political and cultural reaction and response to AIDS. In Uganda this was a highly critical response. "While much has been achieved, there is widespread feeling in Uganda that more could be done to reduce the spread of HIV and tackle its consequences" (unattributed UNDP grey literature, September 1990).

Although nowhere acknowledged, this critical response was surely not unrelated to the exposure of corruption among government officials and an expatriate racket. Ugandan medical researchers began to look back at almost a decade of experience (Serwadda and Katongole-Mbidde 1990). Clinicians in Uganda have pointed out how misleading are the national statistics on AIDS for their country. They have explained that small localized serological surveys have been generalized. The use of averaged figures has led to meaningless scientific conclusions.

Simmering popular anxiety over AIDS research and intervention *per se* were clear indications that something was going wrong on the ground. A need was felt to "Launch an awareness/sensitization program to the public on the importance and use of research in general in order to foster cooperation and improve the quality of information being collected" (Uganda Government 1990:9).

This phase of critical analysis extended to a questioning of the government's responsibilities towards those of its citizens who were sick with AIDS and asked whether specific governmental measures should be taken, forcefully, to criminalize those who were "irresponsible".[8] Our brief field trip to Rakai found the coexistence of both compassion and calls for criminalization.

Within anthropology, considerable credit must be given to Carol Barker and Meredeth Turshen for first setting out the need to set western biomedicine's search for victims—victims to blame for their promiscuous sexual behavior and their social irresponsibility—against a recognition that the conditions under which the AIDS virus gives rise to symptoms of AIDS are "poverty, malnutrition, frequent infection, lack of sanitation, and the indiscriminate use of antibiotics" (1987:51).[9]

It is in the spirit of a call for a more comprehensive and rigorous analytical framing of the AIDS pandemic as problematic that we conclude this essay.

The Moving AIDS Frontier in Hidden Uganda

The critical anthropologist must add to the 1990s study of AIDS both a contextual dimension and historical specificity. In Uganda this requires the recognition of widespread warfare, as in much of Africa, throughout the first AIDS decade. Military activity has thwarted scientific research throughout the continent. Uganda's so-called National Survey of 1989 was, in fact, not carried out in four of the nation's thirteen regions, because it was not safe to enter them. These regions all lay in the north and east of the country.

As AIDS research develops in the 1990s the link must be made more directly with war and famine. The southwest, and particularly Rakai and Masaka districts, were ravaged by warfare during efforts to overthrow the government of Idi Amin (1971-1979). The districts north and northwest of Kampala were laid waste in the guerilla fighting to overthrow Milton Obote's regime (1979-1986) that preceded Museveni's military victory (Furley and May 1989; Hooper and Pirouet 1989). It was during the latter period, in 1982, that the new disease, Slim, was first reported in Uganda.[10]

And what of AIDS reporting from northeast Uganda? In 1986 when the ACP carried out its national survey, only one of 76 healthy adults tested in the rural northeast was infected with HIV (Carswell 1988). A year later a survey of military personnel stationed in the northeast found 30% seropositive for HIV antibodies. (NS 1987). Yet even as late as August 1991 the AIDS intervention programs stopped at Mbalefar, far behind the battlelines of the moving frontier.

How penetrating is likely to be the distribution of AIDS after five years of such conditions? Even more significantly, surely, must we ask, what are the measures being taken for intervention and control on this moving frontier of the epidemic. The question is timely because in Spring 1991 the *Teso Newsletter* in its fifth issue reported that AIDS was "spreading like a bush fire" leaving many orphans (TN 1991:16). The question is one of morality as well as medicine (the subject of our companion paper).

The Museveni government, praised as one of the first in Africa to acknowledge the AIDS epidemic, is only just fully beginning to acknowledge the endemic underdevelopment of those parts of the country where famine conditions breed vulnerability to HIV infection and AIDS. New development plans promise the transformation of rural areas; lawyers' associations and women's organizations work towards eradicating the inequalities that were aggrandized by the administrative exigencies of colonial rule. The problematic of AIDS as primarily a sexually transmitted disease (STD) in Uganda has historical depth as witness the perduring expatriate medical concern with gonorrhea and syphilis throughout Uganda's short eighty year colonial history. A concern barely compatible with the colonial government's expensive provision of advanced medical treatment at Mulago Hospital and its neglect of rural dispensaries and clinics. Whether the AIDS pandemic will be checked in Uganda depends on both the commodification of a medical cure and the striking down of the inequalities likely to hinder its widespread availability.

Conclusion

This chapter has explored the social construction of both history and knowledge centering on the progressive recognition of the magnitude of AIDS as a medical condition of major human and social proportions. By setting out these three paradigms we have sought to reveal the analytic capacities of the social sciences to relate knowledge to practice. The mere fact that paradigms of this type may be readily recognized and that they have social consequences forces social scientists to reflect on the conditions of their engagement in the process of scientific discovery and in formulating and implementing policies.

The chapter traces the shifting focus of social research on AIDS in Uganda from emphasizing curing and caring to more critical analytic frames. Each frame is both an intellectual and empirical construction, relating understanding to practice and knowledge. Initially harnessed to the dictates of a biomedical model, anthropological research was constrained to a narrow and highly focused cluster of problems. Science did not, however, produce the expected immediate cure and thus, the community and its resources were brought into play as a major alternative in providing care for the afflicted. The skills of anthropologists were used to understand community situations related to AIDS. Anthropologists were removed from the complexities of historical and social analysis. The historical and social context of Uganda remained in the background. Context was reduced to event and situation and thus, the processes that had contributed to civil wars, famines, major population dispersals, and the collapse of effective health and welfare services were not fully taken into account. Uganda was treated as of the medical moment, a temporal and spatial frame that began with the recognition of AIDS as a serious medical problem. The final paradigm points to the process of anthropologists restoring historical and social context to events and situations and reasserting their role as critical analysts. Anthropologists cease to be the handmaidens of biomedical experts acting as social epidemiologists scouting out the spread of AIDS among designated high "risk" populations or the parameters of community welfare structures.

It is thus contingent of this chapter that medical conditions are a part only of the context of the AIDS epidemic in Uganda. In immediate terms malnutrition and malaria are indeed far more severe than AIDS. But civil wars and forms of state and group violence have produced dramatic rates of death among the civilian populations of Uganda as they have throughout its history. The central government declared its intention to control AIDS and actively pursued a policy of public education. It has elicited the support of Ugandans, who have taken the message and grounded it in new organizations and patterns of behavior. The 1990s will see the anthropologist researching AIDS in Uganda in the context of religious revival, moral revolution, and Pentecostalism. Uganda as a colonial state was founded on religious interests. Organizational forms that exist in Islam (sensationalized as "fundamentalism") in Catholicism (revered as miracles) and in Protestantism (as Evangelicalism) are living forces in today's Uganda. Then perhaps the voices of Ugandans confronting AIDS will be heard at last.

Notes

1.   The talk on which this chapter is based was given at the New York Metropolitan Medical Anthropology Association, May 8, 1991. We are grateful to our audience on that occasion for their questions and concerns.

2.   Characteristically of popular United States reporting on African affairs, this was said to be after the American Ambassador to Uganda had shown President Museveni "a computerized slide presentation with mathematical models that projected how Uganda would look in the future if nothing was done to stem the AIDS epidemic" (Pelez 1990). Post-colonial studies would suggest a possible racialist denial of rational agency to the African statesman.

3.   This was in contrast with the United States and Europe where most research was conducted among persons with alternative sexual preferences and among drug users. Blood transfusion practices are currently under much scrutiny as yet another point of AIDS transmission. Accounts of the first patients with Slim in Mulago hospital included homosexuals from Rakai district. The point being made is that inquiries that were at first open-ended have become increasingly narrowed in focus to (a) sexual intercourse among (b) heterosexuals.

4.   Most of Christine Obbo's exceptional ethnography of AIDS remains unpublished.

5.   For the unfortunate consequences of this privileging of "traditional" or ethnic culture, see Bond and Vincent 1990.

6.   Our companion essay, "Medicine and Morality," explores the role of the US Baptist Church in combating AIDS in Uganda. For an account of its AIDS Bible in use in Kampala see Chapter 7 of this volume.

7.   See Chapter 7 for an attempt to be analytical.

8.   The "Cuba solution" reported in Chapter 5 of this volume was recently revisited by Scheper-Hughes in a controversial paper at the San Francisco meetings of the American Anthropological Association later published in the association's newsletter.

9.   The spirit of the anti-biomedical movement in anthropology surged up on the last day of the Brunel conference on *AIDS in Developing Countries: Appropriate Social Research Methods* (1990). It was captured in Anne Akeroyd's call for a shift in vision. Her discussions of methods "for whom or for what" (1990a, 1990b) are the most extensive in the field. Themes range from academic neocolonialism to the halo effect of others' unethical practices and racism and her suggestions for future research are, indeed, visionary. See Chapter 2 of this volume.

10. Inquiries into blood transfusions for military personnel in Uganda are at an early stage. There are some indications that companies in California were involved. It is, however, the larger structural picture that we intend to stress. Global and transnational in its infrastructure, it does not seem to us coincidental that cosmopolitical transformations since 1960 (the decade of the break-up of empire in Africa) including the spread of arms, increased non-African expatriate activity, Cold War counter insurgency activities, and the like provide at least a backdrop for the AIDS pandemic. On the other hand, in the long run, none but individuals can be held responsible for organizational responses to these structural trends.

7

Community Based Organizations in Uganda: A Youth Initiative

George C. Bond
Joan Vincent

Introduction

This chapter is intended as a prolegomena to the study of the medico-moral dimensions of AIDS in Uganda. Several issues are involved which we hope to begin to unravel here through our interpretation of the actions of a small organization of students at Makerere University in Kampala in 1988. These include (1) narratives which link beliefs about health and disease to moral and immoral notions of sex; (2) the belief that AIDS and all that follows from it (and precedes it) cannot be contained by official medical explanations, and (3) AIDS in Uganda is an historical event, and, as such, requires processual and historical study: it is a contemporary moment in a much longer history of disease and medicine, morality and material distributions of health and well being in Uganda. The AIDS pandemic in Uganda in 1988 was the historical product of a particular combination of structural forces in its colonial past. This chapter describes the deliberate efforts of a small group of adolescents, college students, to halt the process as they experienced it in the post-colonial present. While it has been recognized that there is need to conduct research into adolescent attitudes and behavior in connection with AIDS (Lindenbaum 1987:59) we know of no other studies that focus on adolescents as self-conscious agents in AIDS intervention in Africa.

The Social and Intellectual Milieu: Uganda in 1988

Most studies of AIDS in Africa deal with state measures, the work of international, non governmental organizations (NGOs) or so-called customary practices. Only the last is primarily concerned with African agency. Inquiry into customary practices is usually carried out either to determine how they constrain biomedical interventions into the pandemic or how they may be harnessed to assist it. Thus in Tanzania and Zambia, for example, "traditional healers" have been recruited by government to help combat the AIDS epidemic in those two countries (e.g. Arkovitz and Manley 1990).

In Uganda biomedical and customary discourses have been encouraged to confront each other at the highest medico-moral level. We attended public fora in which bio-medical practitioners and practitioners of herbal medicine exchanged knowledge and ideas (Bond and Vincent 1988,1991). These were held in one of Kampala's historic hotels and attracted large audiences as well as media attention. Practitioners of herbal medicine whom we met in the field in Rakai district shared the stage with academicians we met in the university in Kampala. This multiplex reality of African medical practice, long recognized by anthropologists (Mitchell 1957), challenges anything but the ideologically constructed bifurcation of the two in the research on AIDS in Africa by biomedical and social science professionals.

Witnessing this very public construction of a Ugandan discourse on AIDS and healing helped us understand a suggestion we received from a well placed government official shortly after our arrival in Kampala that what we should really be studying (as anthropologists) was the politics of the international AIDS community in Uganda. This enactment of consensus by privileged public figures also legitimated the construction of moral-medical intervention for the Ugandan students at Makerere who are the subject of this essay.

In our earliest writing we focussed attention on the rural areas into which AIDS workers—and we ourselves—were catapulted in Rakai district in southwestern Uganda. Later we were able to make private arrangements to conduct our inquiries in the east and northeast of the country, in Jinja and Soroti districts respectively. Not being medical anthropologists, we attempted to situate the AIDS pandemic within the lived experience of the rural populations. In both districts we were obliged to draw attention to the legacy of wars, famines, and migration and the vastly changed social and economic structure of domestic households and communities (both material and constructed/imagined) that has become visible since the mid 1970s.[1] Our field experience of regional differences within Uganda was commonplace to the college students who came to Kampala for higher education from several districts. Their common understanding of lacunae between biomedical knowledge of "traditional" and "customary" practices in their home villages legitimated their organizational effort to intervene in the AIDS prevention campaign that was being mounted by the many national and international bodies then being funded in Uganda. Their "local knowledge" was their justification for action.[2]

Our research between 1988 and 1990 found that few of the persons with whom we spoke in their homes in a range of different rural localities considered AIDS to be of major concern to them—they presented us with a listing of priorities in which health problems were low on the agenda if they appeared there at all.[3] This was in striking contrast to the perceptions and actions of the college students. In taking the initiative to confront the AIDS pandemic in their lives, among their peers, among their kinsmen and in their rural neighborhoods they were making several claims— generational, elite, and national.

This is not the place to provide an account of the relation between systems of medical knowledge and power but we touch upon it in our understanding of the actions of the Makerere students in 1988. They formed a distinct body of interstitial actors between the international medical community and the Ugandan state on the one hand and the rural population on the other. Distinctively, their agency was not that of the official waged or salaried medical or public health worker; it was voluntary and unwaged. Indeed, at the moment they encountered us, meeting by chance but pursuing the opportunity to engage us in their attempt to win some kind of recognition from some kind of authority, their association was little more than a group of like minded young people, men and women, concerned over what *they* could do to counter the spread of AIDS in their country.

Acting out of a sense of moral responsibility for the future of Uganda they were operating in a context of knowledge that configured the AIDS pandemic as an inevitable process of decimation that would leave their nation with no leaders, a lost elite and urban middle class, a destroyed national economy, a missing generation— in short, a cataclysmic view of their universe.

Where precisely in August 1988 had they derived this from? Again, this essay cannot take into account the full paraphernalia of international and governmental reports and professional medical knowledge that set the broad conditions for their particular Ugandan experience. In August 1988 a great deal of this was still held to be confidential and we were pledged not to publicize statistics and graphs. Rivalry (presumably) among government officials and international AIDS researchers involved us in a Kafka-esque scenario in which we were quietly given documents that must not be shared with (presumably) the competition. The AIDS industry was still in the process of taking root in Uganda and not until 1990 was the machinery set up to coordinate the valuable work of national and international scientists, NGOs and funding agencies that in 1988 was still creeping into the tropical daylight as a mildly covert grey literature.[4] In these early days (see Chapter 6) there were good reasons for such control over the dissemination of the biomedical findings about AIDS in Uganda. There was fear of alarming the population at large and fostering an exodus of the professional personnel the capital most needed. There was fear of frightening away non-governmental organizations and investment.

What the students were aware of was the concentration of internationally and government financed professional AIDS-related activities in the Ministry of Health complex at Entebbe, some twenty miles from their university.[5] This was the locale within Uganda for the production and distribution of scientific knowledge of AIDS as it had been for medical and public health research generally in the colonial period. This was the site where institutionalized scientific AIDS knowledge and activity in Uganda was centralized: this was the local hub of governmental and international AIDS activity in the late 1980s.[6]

Visible daily to the college students in the streets of Kampala, and increasingly in the countryside around the capital, were the AIDS vehicles that carried their iconography/ emblems and messages on their sides. If action was being taken against the pandemic, this, the students saw, was how it was being done. Eye-catching posters were then being distributed at various strategic sites—schools and clinics, sports clubs and police stations. In these early days of surveillance and intervention, the eyes they caught were primarily those able to read English or Luganda (later this changed). Both sets of messages—on modern vehicles and public walls—smacked of journalistic headlining or political sound bites. In many places they signified nothing to "the little people," particularly women and those who spoke little English. They successfully grabbed the attention of the English speaking urban elite and were particularly effective with the educated young and adolescent sector of the population. There was, indeed, almost something Yuppie-ish in the AIDS messages in Uganda in 1988.[7]

In this modern African country AIDS is transmitted primarily through heterosexual activity.[8] Paradoxically, in spite of its contemporary, even post-modern form, the AIDS propaganda reflected and disseminated a moral discourse derivative from and heavily influenced by eighteenth and nineteenth century English utilitarian and Christian missionary values. Sexuality was impregnated with the connotation of "sexual immorality."[9] Some of this discourse appeared in local newspapers, especially in letters to the editors in response to this or that scientific revelation or medical advice and reflected non-western values and precepts. Some, as we learned from the college students, was propagated in more exclusive circles of medico-moral distribution, particularly the publications of American and Canadian evangelical churches.

What was the official problematic? The behavior of Ugandans was seen (1) as responsible for the introduction and spread of the AIDS pandemic and (2) as a constraint on policy makers and medical experts. What was the students problematic? How to assert personal agency. Both problematics stemmed from the incontrovertible fact that there is no known cure for AIDS and that the Uganda government had responsibly, publicly and internationally acknowledged the extent of HIV infection in the Ugandan population.

The unexplained but rapid spread of HIV infection and AIDS throughout Africa was common knowledge. One of the pieces of scientifically tracked knowledge made known to us in August 1988 but not available at that time to the general public was the rapid advance of the moving frontier of AIDS within Uganda's international borders. Many of the young men and women of Makerere had already witnessed the deaths from AIDS of their classmates; they were also aware of the "scandalous" gossip about diplomats and high ranking government officials who had left the country to avail themselves (or their children) of the better AIDS treatment facilities in neighboring Zaire. In all of this, one message had communicated itself more powerfully than any other: *the most unfortunate property of AIDS is that human beings themselves are the carriers and only through their own efforts might they attempt to control its progress.*

"Just as disease is a social construction, misinformation is socially constructed too" (Lindenbaum 1987:59). Whether in origin AIDS was a visitation from God or from "Europeans," whether it came about through earlier medical interventions or was acquired from green monkeys (Gilks 1991), its progression, the Makerere students believed, could only be halted through educating the people and encouraging them to change their ways. In this belief, too, of course, they inherited the mantle of the Scottish and English moral philosophers of the eighteenth and nineteenth centuries.

Living with AIDS:
Knowledge and Powerlessness in the Academic Community

Like many African universities Makerere was state funded and concerned to develop programs that furthered the legal, political and economic development of the nation. This had been its brief in colonial times and after its wrenching ordeals during Amin's regime, President Museveni was beginning to rebuild and restore its mission as a regional, continental and, indeed, international educational site of higher learning.

The university and the medical research school had a long historical involvement with public health in Uganda (Beck 1970). Medical records were good in Uganda going back to 1944 and the Medical School had a fine research record. The "discovery" of generalized aggressive Kaposi's sarcoma was made in Uganda in 1962. AIDS was first diagnosed in the USA in 1981 and in Africa in 1983 (Chumeck et al. 1983:642). World awareness of bio-medical and social science research into AIDS in Uganda may be dated from 1985 when David Serwadda of the Department of Medicine of Makerere University Medical School, Mulago Hospital in Kampala and his colleagues published a short article in *The Lancet*, "Slim Disease: A New Disease in Uganda and its Association with HTLV-III Infection" (Serwadda et al. 1985:849-852).

Serwadda and his colleagues reported the first patients as having been seen at Mulago Hospital in 1982. One of the college students with whom we spoke told us of having visited the hospital wards and the clutch of symptoms the <u>Lancet</u> article described would have been familiar to many. By 1988 most would have known at least one sufferer, perhaps a family member, with the ominous signs of diarrhea, wasting, and the dry itchy cough of the HIV infected. Most would have seen infected youths returning to their natal villages from Kampala, perhaps from the college itself, to die among their kinsfolk.

In the hospital setting, most of the HIV infected presented with fever, an itchy maculopapular rash, general malaise, prolonged diarrhoea, occasional respiratory symptoms and oral candidiasis, but the most dominant feature was wasting and weight loss—hence the designation, "Slim". Malaria and sexually transmitted diseases (principally gonorrhea and syphilis) had long been prevalent and widespread in both urban and rural Uganda. Only when wasting and weight loss were highly visible did the sick seek medical or other help.

Dr. Serwadda and his colleagues extracted from Ministry of Health records a typical history found in reports of early cases of AIDS in Uganda. We may interpret this here as the second-hand experience that many of the Makerere students may well have had with AIDS by August 1988. Serwadda's description was as follows:

> In the first six months the patient experiences general malaise and intermittent fevers for which he may treat himself or receive aspirin, chloroquine or chloramphenicol. In due course he develops loss of appetite. In the next six months intermittent diarrhoea starts. There is gradual weight loss and the patient is pale. Most patients at this point in time rely on traditional healers, as to many the disease is attributed to witchcraft. After one year the patient typically develops a maculopapular rash, which is very itchy, all over the body. The skin becomes ugly with hyper-pigmented scars. There may be a cough, usually dry but sometimes productive. By this stage, sometimes earlier, the patient is so weak that, if taken to hospital, not much can be done to help him and death follows (Serwadda et al. 1985:850).

What, in particular, of this experience would most have struck the Ugandan adolescents who took it into their own hands to form an organization to propagate knowledge about AIDS in the villages from which they came?

First, surely the wasting away of the strong male body since, as is common in the language codes of medical scientific knowledge "the patient" is categorically male.[10] AIDS at this early stage appeared to be a disease that struck predominantly at young men: among Ugandans it was young men who traveled in search of work; young men who "used" prostitutes; young men who served in the armed forces; young men who were given blood transfusions for war wounds; young men (mostly) who received scholarships to travel and live abroad. Not until 1990 was the question asked publicly "AIDS and HIV infection in Uganda— are more women infected than men? (Berkley, Naamara, Okware et al. 1990).

Secondly, particularly disturbing to the young college students was the *ignorance* of so many of their uneducated (i.e. un-Western-educated) countrymen of the "causes" of disease (any disease) and their proneness to blame affliction on the actions of their fellows—jealousy, envy, spite—or their own neglect of their deceased ancestors. They would probably have been more tolerant of the behavior of sufferers who turned to local healers than were many of the expatriate biomedical professionals at this time. Nevertheless, their voluntary intervention rested on their superior knowledge of science and it was their mission to educate their less fortunate citizens in the teachings of the modern biomedical profession insofar as they were enculturated in them.

Finally, surely, it is the slow, dragging nature of the disease and the sense that there was no knowing how far it had already progressed either in the bodies they knew or the body politic, that prompted the students to take action, to "put in their oar" in AIDS education/prevention. And why did they believe themselves especially qualified for this task? They were *strong, educated, idealistic, patriotic* young Ugandans.[11]

The students imitated the professional labeling of the international AIDS community and their government in viewing their organization as an "AIDS control" association but its name (which had to be registered with the Ministry of Health) made it clear that it drew explicitly on the university's undergraduate community for its task force. They named it the Makerere University Students AIDS Control Association (MUSACA). As such it contained and expressed multiple understandings of AIDS to be sure but in common among the organizers was a certain disillusion of some students with what appeared to them as an over-reliance on international efforts and their felt need to find "a Ugandan solution".[12]

Highly significant is the fact that the young men and women who formed MUSACA were prepared to confront the intellectual contradictions in their own lives. Whether as catholics, Protestants or Muslims, they were at a conjuncture where western scientific knowledge of AIDS being a sexually transmitted disease co-inhabited with their own "African" sexual norms that were, for the majority of them, legitimated by a "traditional" or "customary" moral code that required pre-marital sexual experiences, sanctioned polygamy in practice if not consistently in principle, and anticipated extra-marital sexual relations for both marriage partners. Ideally, claims to "modern" identity as western-educated university students could resolve the contradiction but practically, knowledge of the actual moral and sexual behavior of similarly western-educated elite members of their society, necessarily clouded their vision. Not "traditional" patriarchy (beloved of social scientists addressing AIDS in Africa) but "modern" power upheld the contradictions. The powerful example of the Roman Catholic church in its condemnation of condom use, a condemnation voiced also by President Museveni himself, did not aid reconciliation.[13] It epitomized rather the contradictions with which the students allying themselves with the biomedical and social science AIDS community were obliged to live.

The young men and women who formed MUSACA were interstitial within Ugandan society in other ways too. As adolescents they were alert to the sickness striking down their kin and peers even as they themselves were embarking on a new (and possibly final prenuptial) phase of wide-ranging adolescent sexual liaisons encouraged and approved within their cultural upbringing. Coming from many different regions within Uganda, they were young men and women engaged in acquiring an enlightened, "Western"-oriented education at the nation's long established university. On graduation, they would be clearly marked as members of the country's elite with national and international, cosmopolitan careers ahead of them. As in the case of most people with privileged educations, "old-school ties" would form the basis of networks that served them well through life.[14] On these various grounds, therefore, it is valuable to assess their self-chosen mode of voluntary organization within Uganda's AIDS prevention program.

A Lost Generation?

An analysis of the cumulative number of AIDS cases reported to the Ministry of Health in May 1988 showed the incidence of AIDS in children age 0-4 of both sexes; a decline in incidence reported for females age 5-12 and for males 5-15; a peaking in both sexes up until age 45; and a gradual decline for both sexes age 45-65. Incidence reported after 65 appeared only in males. Because of this finding, Uganda's national AIDS Control Program focussed its preventive education program on the child cohort (female 5-12; male 5-15). The university students who formed MUSACA were unread in the professional medical findings summarized above and unaware of the government's rationale (in terms of public health expenditure) for adopting this chosen course of action. The students observed what was being done organizationally and for them it was as if their generation had "officially" been given up for lost.

In 1987 the Ugandan government was one of the first in Africa to acknowledge the existence of the AIDS epidemic within its national boundaries and to seek the collaboration of international programs. In May 1987 it organized an international conference in Kampala with the help of the World Health Organization. A National AIDS Control Program was inaugurated (NACP) which has since become a model for such programs in other African countries. Indeed this was but the first of many ways in which the Uganda experience served as a prototype for the "International AIDS package" that was developed, mainly in Britain and the United States, in the 1980s. As we also suggest (Chapter 6) the Ugandan experience must also be read as a cautionary tale.

The technical package introduced in 1987 had seven main components. These were mass public education and information; blood screening and the rehabilitation of the Blood Transfusion Service (badly needed after eight years of intermittent warfare); the protection of the public, health workers and children through the supplying of syringes, needles, gloves, aprons, boots and disinfectants; equipment; and condoms; the establishment of an effective National Surveillance System; the supplying of drugs for the treatment of AIDS cases; the training and orientation of health workers; and, finally, the instigation of Operational Research, both Knowledge, Attitudes and Practices (KAP) studies for health education, and sero-epidemiology and risk factor research. A Five Year Plan was announced calling for the expenditure of US$ 21,500,000. This was the active intervention environment that provided the context of knowledge for the University students who formed MUSACA.

The Students' Voluntary Mobilization for Action

The Makerere University Students' AIDS Control Association (MUSACA) was formed in February 1988. At this time only two districts out of 33 in Uganda had not reported AIDS cases, most reporting between 1 and 100 cases. In only two districts were over 100 cases reported. One was Kampala, the capital city, where

Mulago Hospital and the University were located. Here were 35 per cent of all the cases reported in Uganda; the other district was Masaka in the southwest of the country (23%).[15]

The formal registration of MUSACA as a University student organization required a membership of 35 students and its recognition by the Vice Chancellor. It arose out of the students' concern that the people in their home areas were still ignorant about the causes and transmission of AIDS and their object was to carry what they had learned about it in medical and science courses back to them, teaching from their homes. To this end they approached various international organizations that had come together under the ACP in Uganda to seek funds, particularly to cover transport costs (i.e. fares home and bicycles to use to tour the countryside). By August 1988 when we accidentally encountered association members it had received or hoped to receive assistance from UNICEF, the Education officer of the ACP, and the Ministry of Youth, Culture and Sports. The organizer with whom we first spoke wore in his lapel a MUSACA anti-AIDS button that the association had designed but we failed to inquire into its costing, manufacture or distribution.

In what follows, it is necessary to distinguish between the association's charter and the volunteered initiatives and views of MUSACA's founder and most active organizer. The first took the form of the document stating MUSACA's aims and objectives that they submitted to the Vice Chancellor to win approval. The second we construct from the initiatives and responses of the student organizer as we talked with him about the student movement. Both may be submitted to a texist interpretation. Our own commentary then follows.

Aims and Objectives

To obtain University approval and recognition it was necessary for the students self-consciously to construct a charter for MUSACA. The phrases quoted in the following passage are taken directly from it. Their objectives were set out and enumerated as follows:

1. To set up educational programs, especially in the rural areas, through the two lowest tiers of the government's administrative structure. To launch their campaign in schools, hospitals and other institutions. Special emphasis was to be put on sex education.
2. To eradicate completely fear of AIDS through "enlightenment" and understanding of the disease. This aimed at "the full involvement of all people in matters of national development."
3. To reach a compromise between control measures and the perpetuation of mankind. A sound emphasis was to be placed on "the proper use of sex."
4. To help and nurse the victims as much as possible thus "reducing the trench" between the victims and the society. This was to be done through regular visiting, "preaching," sharing of interests and showing compassion to victims.

5. To stimulate students about humanitarian causes through mobilization. The introduction of resourcefulness and responsibility among the university students was "aimed at brightening the future of Uganda."
6. To be fully involved in both medical and social research about AIDS. The Association was to work both in conjunction with other organizations and researchers and also independently. The ultimate establishment of "a reliable cure for AIDS shall be the goal of the Association."

Commentary

The students saw their mission as combating ignorance about the causes and transmission of AIDS. Among the possible risk factors, as they saw them, in their home areas were "cultural ceremonies" such as initiation rites, certain treatments for headaches which required that incisions be made, often with the use of the same razor blade on several patients. Ear-piercing was also suspect. They were also worried about transmission of AIDS through saliva in beer drinks when reeds (*luseke* or *epi*) or drinking straws were passed from person to person.

The students concern with the mores and customs of their "home areas" reflected the centralization of higher education in Uganda. Most had grown up and received secondary schooling in the rural areas although a few would have attended elite boarding schools near the capital. In dress and behavior these were the New Men, budding professionals, returning only during university vacations to the homes of the rural kinsmen who had financed their schooling. Their personal and political identities remained attached to place; their "enlightenment" was represented by their adoption of English, the national language of Uganda, rather than the vernacular African languages of their "home areas".

We were struck by the extent to which the organizers appeared more concerned with abandoning or modifying "traditional" rural customs than with addressing the problems of disco behavior among young people in towns. In response to our questions, they acknowledged that a lot of "risky behavior" went on in discos, night clubs, and bars. Perhaps a Town/Gown sense of superiority, a sensitivity to class, a sense that since they did not belong to the Town they had no "right" to proselytize there, or simply the procedural difficulty in intervening in urban settings deterred them. In any event, needle sharing in drug use, "prostitution" and homosexuality were not on their agenda.

The students offered Health Education that was, as they put it, "both Scientific and Biblical." The scientific component reflected a three hour lecture on AIDS given in the university; the biblical component taught that "God is one and Medical Science answers questions about AIDS." The primary student organizer continually spoke of their educational efforts as "preaching."

The Makere University Students AIDS Control Association used Bibles published by the United States Baptist Church. These were printed in Great Britain for the International Bible Society and contained, inside the front cover, a two-page spread: on the left hand side, "Medical Science Answers Five Questions Related to

AIDS" and, on the right hand side, "God's Word Answers Five Questions related to AIDS." The bibles were supplied without charge by the Baptists for use in churches of all denominations. The biblical answers were accompanied by texts from the Old and New Testaments. The Mission Bible contains texts that prophesy the advent of AIDS in the world besides supporting the message of the Catholic Church in Uganda replacing the National AIDS Control Program's "Love Carefully" with the Church's preferred "Love Faithfully."

Uganda is a religiously plural society with a population largely divided between catholics and Protestants but with a very large Muslim minority. Struck by the apparently large Christian component in the Association's preaching mission, we asked if Muslim students had joined it. We were told that they formed an "Islamic Unit" within it and that the Imams had welcomed the students' endeavors as a supplement to their own use of the Koran to counter sexual promiscuity and inculcate moral behavior. It may again be noted that the Association's educational goals were directed solely at the heterosexual transmission of AIDS.

Women had made such an advance into public life with the National Revolutionary movement that it was surprising to learn that the association had begun with 35 male and only 5 female students. By mid 1988, however, it had 200 members of whom 50 were women. Apparently, women were, at first, reluctant to associate themselves with the AIDS program lest it be thought that they were women of loose morals (Bond and Vincent 1991). A scandal had broken earlier over some women students and their wealthy "sugar daddies" (the term was used in the Kampala press) whose cars were seen collecting them from the campus dorms.

The students had an elite view of the AIDS arena in which travel to hospitals in Zaire for treatment and the absenting strategies of government ministers' sons and daughters was commonplace. They spoke of AIDS conferences in Stockholm and elsewhere in connection with the finding of new cures. Above all, they were well informed about the Minister of Finance's recent statement about the possible impact of AIDS on the nation's professional middle class (to which they aspired), on the Kampala working class, and thus on the national economy.

The formation of the Makerere University AIDS Control Association provided a bulwark for its members as much against peer pressure as against AIDS. The "looser morals," as they saw it, of those young people who engaged in "promiscuous love making" were sanctioned by an older generation's acceptance of male "grazing" which was in turn sanctioned by "African" custom. Perhaps they too had given up on those of their own generation (whether consciously or not, whether rationally or not) to save the next. The students recognized that AIDS was what they called a "social problem" at the university, students with AIDS falling behind in their studies, infecting female students. They spoke of student suicides in the previous six months.

Climactically, this series of events led them to form their own AIDS control association. Their proposal was simple and their expectations of help were low. They were offering the services of their members during the summer vacation from the university, living at home and proselytizing in their home towns and villages. In return they asked a small salary and a cost of living allowance along with funds to buy bicycles. Their requests were inordinately modest.

Conclusion

The reasons given for the formation of MUSACA reflected the values and attitudes of a section of the young, educated Ugandan upper and middle classes. This was the population category to which most of the Ministry of Health's propaganda about AIDS appeared to be directed in spite of their announced aim of reaching the masses of the people. Most of its posters were in English (the national language of Uganda) and the NACP vehicles which went out into the countryside bore English stickers. In our notebooks, we characterized them as being, apparently, "Yuppie oriented."[16] This was beginning to change in 1988 when we conducted our interviews. Nevertheless, the best known of the AIDS prevention slogans remained "Zero Grazing." This was highly offensive to large sections of the population, including women and the young Catholic students at Makerere. MUSACA, in its goal of reaching out into the home areas of the students, teaching the younger generation and their own less educated elders, was, in part, an effort to provide a more Ugandan, a more nationalistic response to the internationalized crisis.

As a civil war generation, the students were wholly pragmatic in their recognition of the fact that they would only be able to work in the rural areas with the approval of the local administrative power structure. Their initial emphasis was on education and their role as educated persons. Later clauses in their charter (and even more the responses to questions) stressed on caring as well as curing and the need for humanitarianism and volunteerism. In this respect, they reflected an ethos today expressed by many Kampala intellectuals, including those at Makerere University Medical School and Mulago Hospital.

This, too, reflected a climacteric, the critical judgement that, the devastating enemy AIDS having been faced head on, Uganda as a nation must establish itself more distinctively in the ensuing battle against it. The dedication to service of the students who formed the Makerere University AIDS Control Association was captured shortly afterwards by David Serwadda, the Ugandan medical researcher who had co-authored the article in *The Lancet* that first alerted the international community to the new Ugandan disease Slim in 1985:

> It sometimes seems (he wrote) that researchers (and funding agencies) from overseas find it easier than their local colleagues to overlook the suffering caused by AIDS to individuals and communities in Africa.

In this article, again published in *The Lancet* (1990:843), Serwadda and his co-author, E.Katongole-Mbidde, address problems for AIDS research and researchers. They call (1) for a greater service commitment to the local population in western-financed bio-medical studies; (2) for greater recognition of the part played by African collaborators when data is exported to be analyzed by short-contract experts; and (3) for, above all, more sensitivity to the effects of research projects on local study populations.

This appears to us part and parcel of the context of biomedical AIDS knowledge in Uganda shared by the Makerere students. But whereas the MUSACA members saw the problem from the outside looking in, the Ugandan medical researchers had the inside story. Within the history of preventive research a critical moment (a moment of critique) is reached when the scientists and professionals become aware that community response and organization promises to be more effective than campaigns launched by national and cosmopolitan centers. This was the case in the well recorded instances of leprosy control (Pearson 1988) and smallpox inoculation programs. Too often such campaigns fund a universalistic application of centralized programs often on the basis of categorical and statistical social science findings generated out of research in the United States or Europe with vastly different target populations. Often an available technological package shapes the direction that research, education and intervention take.

Uganda is today in the forefront of community based organization in response to the AIDS epidemic in Africa. We suggest that in part this is because of the somewhat bitter phase it reached in the late 1980s as a result of its bio-medical and lived experience with AIDS suffering (Chapter 6). A Ugandan AIDS counseling group, TASO (The Aids Support Organization) was established through voluntary efforts as early as 1986 but there are also smaller, similar, less well known local community initiatives. Some were mounted by women's groups, others by parochial bodies and concerned citizen-carers throughout Uganda. Those organizations that prove most effective are conducted by peers, using a common language, providing knowledge, and based on social interaction other than that which is necessarily HIV or AIDS related.

Something of a chasm lies between a biomedical recognition of an AIDS patient and an anthropological recognition of a person with AIDS. Correctly the former focuses professionally on the diseased body; the latter on the social individual who happens to have AIDS. To counter the rather monocausal type of research inquiry that categorizing and targeting encourages, we have coined the term "multiple contingency risk" (MCR) to describe the situation of certain kinds of AIDS victim in Uganda (Bond and Vincent 1988b). Our present focus on community based organizations—here in the context of elite education but elsewhere within the political economy of family and household in rural areas of Uganda—leads us similarly towards delineating analytically caring and support mechanisms *contingent* on existing and pre-existing social intercourse.

Finally, attention must be drawn to the methodological shortcomings of some social science research on the AIDS epidemic in Africa. There is now a growing literature in Public Health, medical, sociological and anthropological journals on the contrasting qualities of bio-medical and social science research models in Africa; on the hegemonic discourse of the medical community; and the need for more evidence of the impact AIDS is having on people (Akeroyd 1990a, 1990b). Dr. Susan Hunter of Makerere University, a consultant with UNICEF in Kampala responsible for developing an association of non-governmental organizations (NGOs) has written of the need to develop methodologies for data collection and planning that address "the human face" of AIDS in Africa (1990).[17] She argues forcefully that "AIDS research cannot be context poor. To be ethical and methodologically correct, it must be context rich" (1990:9). Like the study of multiple contingency risks, community based organizational studies cannot but be context rich and thus provide a valuable component in a *coherent* strategy for the scientific study of AIDS in Africa.

Notes

1.   Bond and Vincent 1991. We called this essay "Living on the edge" in part because the rural population with which it dealt lived close to the international boundary of southern Uganda, and in part because the impact of AIDS had rendered many households vulnerable to economic and social forces beyond their control. Our methodological focus on spatial "fields of force" and "arenas of action/agency" also negates binary oppositions between traditional and modern, rural and urban, custom and convention.

2.   We follow Foucault 1980 rather than Geertz 1983 in our understanding of "local knowledge."

3.   Bond and Vincent 1991.

4.   In August 1988 this form of "grey literature" was known only to medical personnel and AIDS researchers and made available unevenly among them.

5.   The physical distance between the government departments at Entebbe and the capital at Kampala was also a social distance. On the shores of Lake Victoria, close by the Sailing Club and the Lake Victoria Hotel, the climate at Entebbe was considered more salubrious for "European" settlement in colonial times. An AIDS gap existed in 1988 that placed medical research and treatment at Mulago Hospital (much of its by Ugandan African and Asian medical practitioners) in the Ngambo section of Kampala (close by Makerere University) and the "international AIDS community" (made of mostly but not entirely of Europeans and Americans) in Entebbe. The Makerere student organizer was obliged to hitch lifts in private vehicles to travel the distance between the two.

6.   It was to contrast shortly afterwards with non governmental AIDS agencies and Relief organizations (particularly those concerned with children and famine relief as well as rural development) which located in downtown Kampala.

7.   Bond and Vincent 1988. Uganda Field Report, HIV Center, New York State Psychiatric Institute and Columbia University Presbyterian Hospital (Unpublished. Confidential).

8.   The three main patterns of HIV transmission and manifestation in Africa are (1) heterosexual sexual intercourse; (2) mother to child in pregnancy; and (3) blood transfusions. By 1990 in Uganda, heterosexual contact accounted for over 90% of recorded transmission cases; mother to child transmission accounted for 10%; and blood transmission 1%.

9.   Adam Smith, Thomas Malthus, Jeremy Bentham and Edwin Chadwick stalk, largely unrecognized, in the biomedical moral discourse on AIDS. For a rare explicit acknowledgment of Adam Smith at least, see Trotter 1993:191-2.

10. See Chapter 6 of this volume for the circumstances under which the question was asked.

11. We are familiar with the concept of "War on Want" or "War on Poverty." In postwar Uganda in which victory had lain with the young soldiers of now President Museveni's National Revolutionary Army, the nationalist commitment of the young college students was almost to be taken for granted. The extent of evangelical commitment to a "War on AIDS"is discussed in our essay on morality and medicine in Uganda.

12. This again may well have been related to the feeling that Ugandans were no longer themselves in control of the measures being adopted to educate the Ugandan, their Ugandan, public thereby averting the further spread of the disease.

13. Our questioning about the use of condoms was dismissed summarily as "not applicable" by one Catholic student respondent; the important thing was to have only one sexual partner. This was strongly antithetical to the "mixed messages" conveyed by the international propaganda and, unlike other respondents on the subject, *not* couched in terms of African cultural practice but in terms of Christian principle. Other respondents dismissed condoms as being "not strong enough" for African men.

14. A Ugandan anthropologist, Christine Obbo, has begun to trace AIDS deaths among small clusters within such networks and to explore High School students' attitudes to "elite deaths" (1991b).

15. It must be stressed that these were *reported* AIDS cases. Of these 90% had serum drawn for testing and were sero-positive for HIV-1 antibodies by ELISA. Other cases were reported on the basis of the Uganda clinical case definition for AIDS. Social and behavioral attributes of AIDS cases were not routinely recorded and the data appears to be collected for clinical rather than behavioral analysis. Of the 96% of the cases that recorded gender , 47% were male and 53% female. Mean age for males was 28.7 years and for females 24.6 years. Of the 49% that reported residence, 46% were urban and 54% rural.

16. In our *Uganda Field Report* for the HIV Center for Clinical and behavioral Studies, New York State Psychiatric Hospital and Columbia University (Bond and Vincent 1988a) we discussed five categories of AIDS posters and bumper stickers: (1) colorful Yuppie-type posters; (2) indigenous language leaflets; (3) a UNICEF primary school kit; (4) bumper stickers (seen not on cars but at ACP headquarters) and (5) the anti-AIDS button of MUSACA.

17. Dr. Hunter's path-breaking research on orphans in Uganda is reviewed in Chapter 6.

8

Female Genital Health
and the Risk of HIV Transmission

Regina McNamara

Introduction

Preservation of the intact surface of the female genital tract is an important defense against heterosexual transmission of HIV. If the vaginal epithelial mucosa, the female's normal guard against infection, is not intact when the male deposits infectious semen, susceptibility to HIV transmission may be significantly increased. Sexually transmitted diseases (STD) are one source of damage and their association with HIV transmission is well-documented (WHO 1989, 1990; Wasserheit 1992). Other causes of genital trauma and infection in both women and men that may open a pathway to HIV have been given little attention. For women, cultural conditions and inadequate health services compound the disadvantages of sexual and social inequality to increase their vulnerability to infection and limit their resources for treatment.

This discussion of genital infection and trauma is intended to convey the widespread nature of the problem and its roots in the social and economic context of the lives of women in developing countries. Barriers to diagnosis and treatment of genital conditions are often specific to women, varying in different cultures but with common themes: lack of information, differential access to health care, violation of norms of personal modesty, and a narrow perspective on, ignorance or denigration of women's needs. These barriers can be lowered with education, economic opportunities, better and more available health services, and preventive methods that women can control for their own protection. To accomplish all this, the health and well-being of women must be prominent on national and international research and aid agendas.

Genital Infection and Trauma

In the following discussion it is understood that intact vaginal epithelial mucosa may not be sufficient protection against HIV transmission during intercourse and the presumption of absence of an STD or other genital condition does not lessen the importance of condoms. Study of the action of the virus on cells continues and current knowledge indicates that genital health can decrease although not eliminate susceptibility to infection.

Sexually Transmitted Disease

The term "sexually transmitted disease" extends the list of traditional venereal diseases (gonorrhea, syphilis, chancroid, lymphogranuloma venereum, and granuloma inguinale) to cover more than 20 organisms and syndromes, including chlamydia, genital herpes, and human papillomovirus (HPV) infections. The major primary manifestations of sexually transmitted infections throughout the world include urethritis in men, cervicitis and vaginitis in women, and genital ulcers, genital warts, and enteric infections in both men and women. With infections of the lower reproductive tract, women can experience abnormal vaginal discharge, a burning feeling with urination, abnormal vaginal bleeding, and genital pain or itching.

Studies undertaken in Africa that control for sexual behavior have produced compelling evidence of the association of genital ulcer disease (GUD) caused by syphilis, chancroid, and genital herpes with increased risk of HIV infection (Wasserheit 1992). A WHO expert committee meeting in 1989 concurred that it is biologically plausible for all STD pathogens that cause genital ulcers or inflammation to be risk factors for increased infectiousness or increased susceptibility to HIV (WHO 1989). Although data on STD that are not ulcerative are less conclusive, African women with gonorrhea or chlamydial infection of the cervix, or with vaginal discharge caused by trichomonas have been found to be at higher risk of heterosexual HIV transmission (Aral and Holmes 1991). These infections are far more common than the ulcerative diseases and therefore, if they do facilitate HIV transmission, their effects in the population will be greater (Wasserheit 1992).

Ulcerative STDs are believed to increase susceptibility by disrupting the epithelial barriers in the genital tract. A second mechanism appears to operate through an increase in the normally present lymphocytes and macrophages which occurs with genital tract inflammation. These are HIV target cells and their increase could augment susceptibility to infection.

The prevalence of STD organisms, and thus the patterns of disease, vary greatly among and within world regions and within countries. In Western countries, at present, the herpes simplex virus (HSV) is the most common cause of genital ulcer disease (GUD); in many developing countries, syphilis and chancroid appear to be the most common causes (Hatcher et al. 1994). Rates are approximate since facilities for testing and treatment are scarce in developing countries, private physicians in developed countries frequently do not report their patients' STD, population-based studies are rare, and much of the research is subject to biases inherent in studies of selected groups (e.g., sex workers, STD clinic patients, prenatal and family planning clients).

A female is more likely than a male to be infected from a single act of intercourse with an STD-infected partner. With gonorrhea, for example, the single-event risk for the male is 25 percent; for the woman it is 50 percent (Hatcher et al. 1994). Yet women are seriously undercounted in STD data in all countries, in part because their conditions are often asymptomatic, but also because services they can or will use are not available. Clinical diagnosis and screening for infection are rarely included with services offered at family planning, antenatal, or maternal and child health (MCH) clinics. STD clinics, where they are available, are usually geared to the treatment of men and are not acceptable to women. Consequently, estimates of the gender distribution of the incidence of STD cannot be made with any confidence.

An international review of research on female reproductive tract infections found greater prevalence in African studies than those conducted among Asian or Latin American populations. The median of the rates of gonorrhea found in the studies in African countries was 10 percent. The median of rates was 1 percent for the Asian studies, and 6 percent for the Latin American studies. Median rates of trichomoniasis were 19 percent, 11 percent and 12 percent for African, Asian and Latin American studies, respectively (Dixon-Mueller and Wasserheit 1991; Wasserheit 1989).

Since the major immediate causes of infertility in women are probably gonorrhea, chlamydia, and other reproductive tract infections, infertility serves as an indirect measure of STD prevalence. Untreated, these infections lead to pelvic inflammatory disease, which leads to tubal inflammation, damage, or distortion, which leads in turn to inability to conceive or to spontaneous abortion (Sherris and Fox 1985). The measure of female infertility used in most population studies is childlessness at the end of the reproductive years, although this incorrectly assigns all childlessness to female infertility rather than male, and misses infertility after first or later births. The indices vary widely, from as low as 1.0-1.5 percent in Korea and Thailand to as high as 13 percent in urban areas of Colombia and 23 percent in one rural area of New Guinea (Belsey 1980).

In sub-Saharan Africa, the highest levels of childlessness have been found for the most part in three zones: Southwestern Sudan and Northwestern Zaire; Cameroon and Gabon; and Southeastern Angola and Northeastern Zambia. These areas, and regions in Burkina Faso and Uganda, have reported over 21 to 40 percent infertility levels. In adjacent areas, levels of childlessness are still well above the 3 percent which is considered a normal benchmark for natural fertility populations (Frank, 1983). A large multi center study conducted by the World Health Organization found tubal occlusion, often resulting from STD, was a cause of infertility in 11 percent of infertile women from developed countries; 49 percent from African countries and 16 percent from other developing countries (cited in Hatcher et al. 1994). Differences in the prevalence of STD, or in access to treatment, may well explain much of the observed differentials in infertility rates.

Genital Trauma

STDs are a major but not the sole source of damage to the female genital tract. Additional sources of infection or trauma that could damage the epithelial barrier include female genital mutilation, childbearing, insertion of objects into the vagina, and trauma during sexual intercourse. Maintaining cleanliness of the genital area under the harsh conditions of nomadic life, drought, or life-long water scarcity requires heroic measures and infections probably caused by inadequate cleansing of cloths used to absorb menstrual blood are reported (Wasserheit et al. 1989).

Female genital mutilation is a plausible cofactor for HIV transmission which has not been adequately studied. Of the three types of operations performed on young girls, the gravest is infibulation, also called pharaonic circumcision. The clitoris, labia minor, and parts of the labia major are removed and the two sides of the vulva are fastened together, leaving a small opening for urination and menstruation. Consequences of infibulation such as inflammation of the genital area, partial closure of the vaginal orifice, abnormal anatomy or friable scar tissue are conditions that, according to the World Health Organization, may increase susceptibility to HIV (WHO/GPA 1990). Long-term sequelae of infibulation known to occur are chronic urinary retention, urinary tract infections, incomplete healing and excessive scar tissue (or keloids) which can cause vaginal obstruction. Childbirth (when the infibulated section is cut open for passage of the infant) can be severely traumatic with consequences as grave as rupture of the vagina. Complications caused by these female genital operations are not reported with any regularity, in part because of the reluctance of the women to expose their genitals for medical examination (Gordon 1991).

In North Sudan, according to preliminary reports from the Demographic and Health Survey, 82 percent of the married women had undergone pharaonic circumcision. An additional 15 percent of the married women underwent Sunna circumcision, the "mildest" form in which the tip of the clitoris is removed, or an intermediate type of excision when the whole clitoris and often adjacent parts including the labia minora are removed (Ahmed and Hamad 1990). The intermediate and Sunna forms are practiced more widely in sub-Saharan Africa and the Middle East than is the pharaonic (which is reported mainly from Ethiopia, Southern Egypt, Somalia and other Red Sea coastal areas). Current estimates of the total number of African women who have undergone some form of circumcision or infibulation approach 100 million (Women's International Network, n.d.).

The Safe Motherhood Initiative launched in Nairobi in 1987 brought to the fore of international discussion the problems of maternal mortality in developing countries. Research and interventions have focused on the risk of death, yet at each delivery the woman confronts risk to the integrity of the genital tract. Tears or incisions during childbirth, with potential for infection, are common traumas of childbirth and massive infections can result from induced or spontaneous abortions. Very young women (especially when childhood nutrition has been poor, infections are frequent, and growth is stunted) are especially vulnerable to risks associated with delivery. Childbirth at very young ages is not a rare event. In Mauritania, for example, 15 percent of the girls have given birth by age 15; in Bangladesh, 21 percent have had at least one child by age 15 (United Nations, 1991:59).

When the pelvis is immature or underdeveloped, cephalopelvic distortion and prolonged obstructed labor can cause damage as severe as vesico-vaginal fistula (VVF). With VVF, there is an opening between the urinary bladder and the vagina and the afflicted women continuously leak urine, wetting their clothes and excoriating their mutilated vulvae and vaginas. Reports on VVF from Pakistan, Turkey, Sudan, Kenya, India, Nigeria, South Africa, Egypt, and Ghana indicate obstetric causes for 80 to 100 percent of the cases identified (Tahzib 1989). In one Nigerian hospital, 30 percent of the VVF cases were under age 15; 59 percent under age 18 (Ampofo et al. 1990). The number of women with VVF is not known; many are believed to be suffering quietly out of sight, shunned as pariahs by family and community and without protection.

Other causes of genital trauma abound, and include traditional practices such as the "gishiri" or "salt cut" in Nigeria which involves incision of part of the interior vaginal wall by a traditional birth attendant, traditional healer, or occasionally by the woman herself. The purpose is to cure a variety of vaginal conditions and infertility (Adebajo 1989).

Herbs, traditional preparations and foreign objects inserted into the vagina can cause inflammation, abrasions and infections, and so increase risk of HIV transmission. Practices may be intended to increase the male partner's pleasure during intercourse. Among pregnant women studied at a hospital clinic in Malawi, 12 percent reported using one or more of the following to tighten the vagina: herbs, aluminum hydroxide, cloth, and stones (silica gel, potassium permanganate, pumice-like stone). Not surprisingly, stones were found to have an irritating and erosive effect on vaginal mucosa and the data reported suggest that they may facilitate entry of HIV (Dallabetta et al. 1990).

Globally, women are known to insert objects into the vagina for medication and especially for contraception or to induce abortion. The array of things used for those purposes in Mexico, for example, includes herbs, pills, soap, and lime (Shedlin and Hollerback 1981). A more complex process is described in Nigeria:

> To prepare [the abortifacient] leaves and seeds from certain local trees (ejirin seeds and itu leaves) are ground and the juice from another tree (epin) added to form a paste. The paste is then made into small balls and dried. As they become dry, more juice is added two or three times. The balls are inserted into the vagina and, according to our informants, they have the effect of destroying the foetus (Adebajo 1989:14).

A cross-cultural study of indigenous fertility regulation conducted in seven countries illustrates the diversity of potentially damaging objects (Newman 1985). In Afghanistan, women reported intravaginal insertion of wooden spoons or sticks treated with copper sulphate to cause heavy bleeding and abortion (Hunte 1985). Egyptian women use aspirin, lemon juice, black pepper and plant stems (Sukkary-Stolba 1985). In other countries, bamboo leaves, grass, the midrib of the coconut palm, water pumped under high pressure, hangers, knitting needles, and umbrellas are abortifacients (Ngin 1985; Low and Newman 1985).

Genital conditions conducive to HIV transmission may also result from sexual intercourse especially in the absence of foreplay when the unlubricated surface is irritated by penile penetration. Among older women, atrophic vaginitis may cause mucosal tears during sexual intercourse (Peterman 1990). Vaginal barrier methods for contraception or STD prevention, discussed below, generally involve use of a spermicide which may cause local irritation of vaginal and cervical tissue (Hatcher et al. 1989).

Damage to the female genitalia and increased susceptibility to HIV infection can result from rape or other forms of violence in sexual intercourse. This is a risk factor especially for sex workers who have repeated encounters with drunk and violent clients. In a Harare, Zimbabwe study, half the sex workers interviewed said that their most recent client was drunk (Wilson et al. 1989). An additional genital hazard comes with the use of condoms for frequent acts of intercourse in a short time period. According to recent reports from focus groups with sex workers in Thailand, the customer with a condom takes a longer time to ejaculate, the lubricant wears off, and friction and irritation follow (Sittitrai et al. 1989; Pramualratana 1994).

Women on average are infected at younger ages than men and, as the epidemic develops and adolescent girls are sought as sexual partners in the belief that they are free of HIV, the gender differential becomes ever more acute. In one region in Uganda, for example, up to 50% of 13 to 18 year-olds are infected compared to 10% of males in that age group (Wawer 1994). In one year, five females per 100 person years and no males seroconverted among 15 to 19 year olds (Wawer et al. 1994). The differential may have physiological causes in addition to those related to gender roles. Among possible explanations are thinner tissue lining the vagina of adolescent girls, providing less protection and more easily damaged; less profuse vaginal mucus; and the exposure of a transition zone of cells that ring the opening of the cervix which moves to a less exposed position in mature women (UNDP 1993).

Diagnosis and Treatment: The Obstacles

Recognizing the major role played by the integrity of the female and male genitalia in reducing heterosexual transmission of HIV can be an important contribution to global prevention efforts, but diagnosis and treatment are possible only when women and men can present themselves to someone with the skills and means to correctly identify their conditions and supply appropriate medications.

Utilization of Health Services

Little is known about utilization of health services by women in developing countries for their own needs. They are usually questioned only about their use of services that are related to reproduction or for their children. The major recent source of information on use of services during pregnancy are the Demographic and Health Surveys conducted in Third World countries in the 1980s and 1990s. These surveys indicate that many women interviewed had at least one visit to a trained midwife or physician at some time during pregnancy, but far fewer delivered with trained assistance. In Egypt, for example, 42 percent of the rural women receive some prenatal care from a physician or trained nurse or midwife; only 19 percent deliver with trained assistance. Seventy-eight percent of rural women in Ghana have at least one prenatal visit; 29 percent have trained assistance at childbirth. In rural Guatemala and Mali, less than 20 percent have trained help at delivery and percentages with prenatal care are scarcely greater. In all countries, urban women are more likely than rural women to use services and strong upward trends in utilization are seen as women's educational levels rise from no education to secondary school. The increase is from 18 to 86 percent for prenatal care in Guatemala, for example, and 27 percent to 95 percent in Mali (Gallin et al. 1993).

Distance from home to the health facility, lack of transportation and lack of funds undoubtedly explain some of the births not attended by trained personnel, yet the differential between source of care for prenatal visits and deliveries also suggests that deliberate choices are being made. The value given to a natural and familiar setting and the spiritual and material support for the woman offered by traditional birth attendants strongly influence a decision to give birth in the home community (Twumasi 1987). These factors weigh heavily against the lack of privacy, unfamiliar positions taken for delivery, shame at crying out before others in a health facility, and the indignity of exposure (Auerbach 1982; Rehan 1984; Schuler et al. 1985; Beeson et al. 1987; Kerns 1989).

The statistics on utilization do not take into account the quality of care (training and skills of the provider, shortages of supplies or equipment such as specula or gloves for internal examinations). For the usual prenatal examination, the woman is weighed, blood pressure is taken, the abdomen may be palpated, urine may be tested, and sometimes blood may be drawn for testing. The woman may be asked about vaginal discharge, itchiness or other symptoms, but a pelvic examination is not always performed if it is not indicated by her history or condition. Even a woman using a modern family planning method, unless it is an IUD or tubectomy, might not be examined internally.

Women often are not aware of the vaginitis and cervicitis which are the common syndromes for lower tract infections (Hatcher et al. 1994). Estimates of asymptomatic conditions range from 10 to 50 percent of women with trichomoniasis, 25 to 30 percent with gonococcal cervicitis, and probably over 50 percent of women with chlamydial cervicitis or bacterial vaginosis (Wasserheit et al. 1989, citing Holmes et al. 1984). Symptoms such as vaginal discharge may be taken to be a fairly normal condition, not requiring medical attention. The discharge and even a substantial degree of discomfort are often ignored (McFalls and McFalls 1984; Orubuloye et al. 1990). In a study conducted in southwestern Uganda, vaginal discharge was reported by 7 percent of the female participants but was observed in 68 percent during clinical examination (Mulder et al. 1992).

Access to Health Services

Differences between men and women in access to health care are acute when conditions are affecting sexual organs. A man with symptoms might go for STD treatment, at least at an advanced stage; his wife is more likely to remain untreated. This is not always because women are unaware of what is happening to their bodies. It can be because their bodies are not seen as requiring care or because cultural values restrict their access to services.

Female doctors are rare in rural areas throughout developing countries and in Moslem cultures especially women may not be examined by a male doctor. Women are often not spared from household and childcare duties to keep clinic hours or to wait at hospitals or dispensaries. Distances to health facilities can be extremely burdensome and travel outside their immediate community may be forbidden to women (Kloos 1987), or inhibited by lack of education and the confidence needed to deal with the official systems. More efficient means of transportation—such as bicycles, motorbikes, horses and donkeys—may be used only by males (Stock 1983).

Where they are confined to purdah, as in Hausa society, a woman must obtain the permission of her husband before leaving the home compound. Many men are reluctant to allow their wives to make long, unescorted journeys for health care, particularly if the husband perceives the wife's illness to be non-threatening and amenable to traditional treatment (Stock 1983).

Men are often the intermediaries between women and health services and assessment of the severity of a condition and the choice of an appropriate source of treatment, if any, may be made by the husband or by senior members of the family. Janzen (1978) found in Zaire that the sufferers retain decision-making rights only if they are adult, capable of walking and traveling, financially able to pay for care and, usually, male.

The obstacles many women face in access to health care have among their causes poverty, lack of education, inferior position in society, and inadequate health systems. One consequence is that they may pass through their entire lives and bear their children, yet never experience an internal examination.

Personal Modesty

Even if symptoms are recognized, and even if services are available, forbidding obstacles to care remain. For women, a strong deterrent is reluctance to undergo a pelvic examination. This was emphatically demonstrated by a survey on female genital operations in the Sudan. Ninety-five percent of the sample population (3,210 women) were interviewed, but only 12 of the women were willing to be examined (Gordon 1991). Some of the women may have wished to conceal the evidence that they had undergone mutilation; the majority were more likely to be expressing their strong sense of personal modesty.

Reluctance to expose the genitals is not unique to women in developing countries. In the United States, for instance, fear of a pelvic examination was cited by 25 percent of adolescents queried as to their reason for not coming sooner to a clinic for family planning (Zabin and Clark 1981). As Scrimshaw states emphatically: "Any woman from just about any culture who has ever had a pelvic examination knows how undignified and embarrassing it feels" (1973:10).

Embarrassment or shame has particular force in some cultures, evidenced by the unpopularity of contraceptive methods that require genital exposure and contact. Injection, for example, has been recommended for women in India so that they might avoid both the mortifying experience of exposure to medical scrutiny and the need to handle their genitals when using a method (Marshall 1973). Embarrassment with genital exposure associated with IUD insertion is reported from Indonesia where the Islamic religion plays a major role in choice of contraceptive method. Many Moslems object to the intimate physical contact between IUD providers and their clients, despite recent rulings from high Moslem councils conditionally endorsing IUD use (Molyneaux et al. 1990).

Modesty as a value central to the image of womanhood is notable in the care taken to cover the genitals of females even in infancy, as in Latin America, while male children are free to expose their genitals until they approach puberty. Douches and coitus-dependent contraceptive methods which violate standards of modesty are rarely used by women in Colombia (Browner 1985) and never among the Aguarunas in Peru who interpret any viewing or manipulation of female sexual organs as erotic (Berlin 1985). Some Mayan women in Guatemala do not remove their skirts even for childbirth (Beck 1991). Mexican women asked to name the parts of their bodies could find no word for the vagina except "la parte" (the part) and that was uttered with manifest embarrassment (Shedlin 1982).

The depth and force of modesty is exemplified by the pregnancy and childbirth practices of rural Hausa/Fulani women in the northern region of Nigeria. Muslim women (in purdah) do not openly admit to their pregnancies. They often labor alone in their compound (with other women keeping within hearing distance in case assistance is required). The traditional birth attendant is called in after the child is born to cut the cord and look after the mother and baby (Sokoto Maternal Health Project 1990).

Fear and stigma surround problems relating to the sexual organs and women suffer in silence. In India, inhibitions about drawing attention to the body can be so great that even female health workers must rely upon verbal accounts of the symptoms of women who will not subject themselves to a physical examination (Ramasubbam 1990).

Feelings of "verguenza," or shame, and their influence on attendance at family planning clinics, were examined by Scrimshaw in detail (1973). Many of the women interviewed in Guayaquil, Ecuador, who never undressed completely before their husbands, were forced to expose themselves to male doctors at the clinic without even a drape over their legs during the pelvic exam. With a drape, at least the woman cannot see the doctor and has some illusion of privacy.

Moroccan women report feeling inhuman when they are ordered to take off their pants and sit in a drafty hall where people walk by while they are waiting to see the service provider for family planning (Mernissi 1975). This study, the Scrimshaw work also from the 1970s, and a much earlier one by Stycos in Puerto Rico (1955), gave serious and scientific attention to a subject that is still acutely and universally felt by women, still a grave problem, and still for the most part ignored.

Sexual Inequality and Stigma

Restrictions on travel, fear of pelvic examination and violation of the sense of personal privacy are sufficient as formidable barriers without the stigma of a sexually-related disease. An association of STD and promiscuity, references to STD as "the woman's disease" in popular parlance in some languages, and common use of the term "reservoirs of infection" to describe prostitutes place the onus solely on the female regardless of the male's multiple relationships. Research in Zaire found that when men are infected, their wives are suspected of infidelity; when women are infected, they are assumed to have "strayed" (Schoepf, cited in Bledsoe 1989:11). The image of women as the source of disease is reinforced by the media and public health announcements, as in the Zambian advertisement "Avoid AIDS. Take Time to Know Her" (Bledsoe 1989:11).

Counseling women about prevention and the need for treatment of their partners may presume incorrectly that they are free to discuss sex and condom use without jeopardy. Yet discussion of this emotionally charged topic is rare in many cultures. A survey of spousal communication in Asian countries, for example, found that close to a third of the women interviewed in the Philippines never talked to their husbands about sexual matters, nor did 47 percent in Singapore or 53 percent in Iran (UNESCAP 1974). Caldwell et al. (1989) comment that in sub-Saharan Africa, sexual activities are rarely discussed either between spouses or between the generations. In Latino culture also, communication between men and women (or parents and children) regarding sex is not the norm (Worth and Dooley 1990; Santos-Ortiz 1990). Folch-Lyon (1981) found, in a study of decision making on the use of family planning in Mexico, that 35 percent of the survey sample had never discussed the subject of birth control with their spouse. In focus groups, women expressed the difficulties they experienced in any discussion of sexual relations with their husband. Castro de Alvarez (1990) observed that cultural norms in their patriarchal society dictate that Latinas appear naive about sexual matters; that a woman knowledgeable about and prepared for a sexual encounter is considered a loose woman. It is thus very difficult to realize the necessary conditions for introducing condom use and persuading a partner to be treated for a STD; that is, relative sexual equality between men and women, the possibility that other sex partners can be acknowledged, and options other than motherhood to define self-identity or self-esteem (Worth 1989).

When there is no communication about sex, and when women fear that their relationships will be jeopardized by asking for safe sex practices, condom promotion among women is likely to fail. The anger at being made to feel responsible for men's sexual behavior expressed by women in a New York City study probably has near universal application. Since "the men decide what is going to happen sexually," if the staff want the men to wear condoms, they have to talk to the men (Worth 1989). Prevention strategies that place the onus on women ignore the subordinate position of the many who are economically and emotionally dependent on their male sexual partners. For these women, negotiation, even perhaps discussion, is not an option (Maldonado 1990).

Among the sociocultural and psychological constraints to overcome in promoting condom use in Zaire cited by Schoepf et al. (1988a), are strong beliefs and feelings about the contribution of semen to women's health and the importance of reproduction. The decision to use a condom is a decision not to be able to reproduce at that time as well as to prevent infection. The general use of condoms may, therefore, be in direct conflict with the desire of women to fulfill their reproductive roles and, with the expectations of their partners and families that they do so. It is also a decision which must be made for each act of intercourse. Women must repeatedly address the issue of sexual decision-making and sexual control, and each time this is done they are emotionally, sexually, physically, and economically vulnerable (Worth 1989).

Summary and Discussion

The causes of damage to the epithelial barrier against vaginal transmission of HIV are numerous: STD, insertion of objects into the vagina, trauma during sexual intercourse, and genital mutilation practices, among others. Also numerous are obstacles to prevention, diagnosis and treatment. Most are embedded in the cultural and economic context of women's lives, to be overcome only with concerted effort on the levels of the local communities and national health systems, and if they have priority on national and international research and aid agendas.

Recommendations in this section are given with the caution that change in women's knowledge, attitudes and behaviors are necessary for their protection, but women do not carry alone the responsibility for prevention of HIV transmission. Men, in their political and economic positions of power as well as their sexual partnerships, are responsible for change that permits women to exercise the control over their bodies and their lives which is their primary protection against HIV (Hamblin and Reid 1991; Carovano 1990).

Community Level

On the level of the local community, the starting point for education of women and men is the message that it is not only for childbearing that women's health is important. Knowledge about their bodies, ability to speak of reproductive organs and processes without shame, hygienic practices—especially for management of menstruation—signs and symptoms of genital-urinary problems must be communicated through social networks in the community. By whatever means, women must be helped to talk of these things together in their own idiom, without embarrassment, to talk with their children, and to help each other devise strategies for raising these issues with men. Men must be helped to be at ease speaking of women's reproductive systems, with women and with each other, candidly but not crudely. Role models must come forth who in their knowledge of and attitudes toward women exemplify a cultural reconstruction of masculinity.

Knowledge about reproductive biology in many societies is transmitted by older experienced women, especially where social separation of sexes emphasizes communication between women rather than between partners (Newman 1985). The local setting may suggest other rules for discussion of sexually-related matters, as in Tunisia where Huston (1978) found that women would never speak of family planning with their daughters or with anyone of a different age group. Yet indigenous women's groups are a near universal resource and women can use them to learn to communicate across generations about genital health and its preservation in their own way, according to their own customs.

Preferences for local, familiar, and predictable midwifery services for childbirth suggest a role for traditional midwives in developing awareness of threats to genital health and the ability to recognize symptoms of STD and advise on resources for treatment. Training traditional birth attendants (TBAs) for safe delivery practices and health education is a fairly widespread practice. Although the trainers usually discourage midwives from performing internal examinations, in order to avoid infections, and their curriculum do not usually cover STD and other genital conditions, midwives can be trained to ask about symptoms, to advise, and, when linked to a health service system, to refer for diagnosis and treatment.

Research on traditional medicine rarely is specific as to conditions that motivate women to seek care, other than pregnancy, although the evidence generally supports the view that traditional practice addresses a broad range of women's conditions. Traditional medicine co-exists with modern medical practice, and it is not uncommon for consultations with both systems to occur serially or concurrently (Janzen 1978; Cosminsky and Scrimshaw 1980; Heggenhougen 1980; Green and Makhubu 1984; Cleland and van Ginneken 1988; Good 1988; Ingstad 1990).

In Malaysia for example, two regional traditional systems (Ayurvedic and Chinese) and the local Malay folk medical system are interrelated as parts of a general Malaysian cultural and social situation, linked on the level of the folk community to the official health system and used widely as additions or alternatives (Heggenhougen 1980). A Guatemalan plantation population can have simultaneous recourse to folk curers (curanderos), herbalists, midwives, spiritists, shamans, injectionists, pharmacists, private physicians, public and private clinics and hospitals, and home remedies (Cosminsky and Scrimshaw 1980). Good (1988) estimates that most African rural areas have at least one part-time traditional healer for every 200 to 300 people; in the towns, one healer for every 400 to 800 people. In Swaziland, at least 85 percent of the population are believed to make use of the services of traditional healers (Green and Makhubu 1984). Many of these opinion leaders and therapists are female. While the usefulness of a traditional healer in communicating information on genital health and its protection would certainly not be universal, this ubiquitous and influential resource should not be overlooked.

Health Systems

Strengthening service systems for prevention and treatment of genital infections and other conditions must be a major national and international priority that should not respect traditional alignments of service categories. The narrow focus of public health programs concerned with women is apparent in their labeling as Maternal and Child Health services. Their rationale lies in the belief that improving women's health is an important precondition to child health and a recent variant of this reasoning focuses on the woman as a potential transmitter of HIV to her infant and as caregiver for AIDS patients and orphaned children. The health systems reflect this limited view of women's lives and potential and the pervasive gender inequalities which deny women control over their own bodies. Expansion of the concept of women's health to encompass the breadth of their activities and concerns is an immediate public health responsibility. Grants for study and research, support for networks of organizations, forums, training, policy analysis, advocacy, and new and improved programs are all required to bring attention to the restrictions on the health services women are now offered—restrictions not only because they are scarce in many places but because of the boundaries they place on women's needs.

Prenatal services offer at least one chance for health care providers to counsel women on protection of the genital tract and to diagnose and treat genital-urinary tract infections. Training of personnel for clinical alertness to adverse genital conditions is necessary; equally necessary are respect for the patients' sense of inappropriate or shameful exposure and care to ensure privacy to the maximum degree possible. Screens constructed from local materials, drapes made from local cloths to shield exposed areas, minimum time without full clothing—these are in themselves indications of concern for feelings as well as relatively simple measures to make services more acceptable to women. Increasing the supply of female medical personnel on all levels is essential. In the prevailing absence of educational opportunities for women from the earliest grades through university degrees, individual women must be assisted with scholarships.

Much of the work needed does not require advanced training. Extensive employment and in-service training of local women in health centers and the community can reduce barriers while it extends the availability of services. Primary health care and family planning services have amply demonstrated the value of paramedical personnel drawn from the local population and trained. Coupled with genuine community participation, especially of women's organizations, in facility and service planning there is then hope that needs, perceptions, problems and expectations can be freely expressed and respected.

Family planning providers can be leaders in the formal sector to explore how the services can reduce the institutional obstacles women encounter. Their programs would be natural providers of services for diagnosis and treatment of genital lesions, inflammations, and infections and they may be the only available source of health care for sexually active women, especially poor women. Substituting modern contraceptives for objects damaging to the vagina (which will also diminish their use as abortifacients), educating patients about risks, diagnosing, treating, counseling about simultaneous treatment for sex partners—these are functions that would be relatively easy to integrate into family planning services, given appropriate training and supplies, and a commitment to reproductive health that extends beyond contraception.

The reality of scarce resources for health care throughout the Third World is glaringly evident in the shortages of laboratories and supplies for diagnosis and medication for treatment of STD. In the shorter time frame, rapid expansion of laboratory testing will not be feasible. It is feasible to develop and subsidize distribution of supplies for inexpensive, relatively simple diagnostic techniques using cervical swabs, vaginal KOH odor, and dipstick assessment of vaginal pH, as demonstrated in a study of reproductive tract infections in Bangladesh (Wasserheit et al. 1989). As appropriate tests are developed, the health systems must undergo the changes necessary to maintain a dependable supply of drugs for treatment as a logistic priority.

Research and Aid Agendas

Priorities for research on female genital conditions are not easily set with a topic so seldom examined in its personal and social complexity. Technological advances and the support of international agencies to make inexpensive diagnostic tests available for Third World women is an obvious and urgent need. Female providers in traditional and modern sectors must be trained to educate, diagnose and treat, and their work must be evaluated through operations research.

Spermicides and diaphragms as barriers have the potential to shift the locus of control over prevention to the women, a preference demonstrated by women who were given the choice in studies in Rwanda (Allen et al. 1989), Ghana and Cameroon (Spieler 1990). As Stein (1990) observed, barriers that depend on the woman alone may be less efficacious than condoms yet be more effective in the long run, if they are consistently and widely used and the condom is not.

Laboratory and clinical studies have indicated that vaginal spermicidal contraceptives which place a chemical barrier between infected fluids and vulnerable mucous membranes may offer women protection against some STD (See

North 1990 for a literature review; Rosenberg and Gollub 1992, for a review of selected studies; and Cates, Stewart and Trussell 1992, for a commentary.) Nonoxynol-9 (N-9), the most widely used spermicide, has been tested, among others, as an HIV virucide and laboratory findings suggest that N-9 offers some protection, but it has not been determined whether spermicides alone, without any mechanical barriers, protect against HIV. Problems encountered in interpreting results of clinical studies have stemmed from selection of special populations (e.g., prostitutes with rates of sexual activity far exceeding the general population) and confounding factors such as high concentrations of N-9 which irritate the genital epithelium and use of N-9 with a vaginal sponge which could itself cause micro lesions.

Female condoms (e.g., pouches made of polyurethane or latex) are available, although they are not yet in a form or at a price that is likely to have wide acceptability. The dilemma or paradox of relying on the male condom as the main strategy to prevent women from HIV transmission stems, of course, from the reality that it is a strategy for men. Since it has little applicability in the context of male-female relationships where the male is dominant and resistant, female-controlled means of mechanical and chemical barrier protection must be identified and rigorously tested, those that are effective must be distributed widely at little or no cost, and they must have appeal to women.

A vaginal virucide which would offer protection against transmission without preventing conception is a vital consideration for women who desire children, and often need to have them in societies where their status and economic security depend upon procreation (Stein 1990). One avenue for research is the possibility that concentrations of N-9 lower than recommended as a spermicide may be effective as a virucide (Stein and Gollub 1991). The urgency of the need to investigate virucides and to develop methods women can use cannot be overstated.

The literature on a possible association of female mutilation with HIV transmission is sparse and speculative. Infection due to mutilation and subsequent trauma, and blood transfusions necessitated by excessive bleeding at childbirth, are plausible routes. The universality of the practice in some African regions suggests that there may be an "at risk" group of appalling dimensions as the epidemic expands geographically. Vigorous investigation of the relationship between female mutilation and HIV transmission must be undertaken.

Societal Transformations

The place of women in society is a primary cause of exposure to risk of HIV infection and a primary barrier to use of health services. Little or no information, restrictions on movement outside the local community, fear of strange environments that are often with justification perceived as hostile, and the male role as mediator between the women and the health system are some of the consequences of women's position discussed in earlier sections of this paper. The changes that must be made in the legal, economic, and cultural spheres over the long term are immense and are largely to be made by those who are favored by the present inequities; over the short term there are collective actions women can take in their local communities. Women together are learning to develop strategies for communication with their sexual partners about HIV, STD, use of condoms, and other sexual behaviors—finding as well the courage and determination to face opposition. Collectively, women are developing strategies to stand up to the official systems, to change men's behavior, to teach and to protect their young daughters, and to realize the strength of unity for survival. They must be assisted with information, with legal aid, with health services, and with opportunities for education and economic independence. A woman's lack of control over the resources for her own physical and mental health and well-being is a violation of human rights that constitutes a direct threat to her life.

9

The Point of View: Perspectives on AIDS in Uganda

Maryinez Lyons

Introduction

In Uganda, a wide spectrum of conceptualizations of HIV/AIDS has emerged as different social groupings struggle to comprehend and cope with the disease.[1] AIDS in Uganda, as elsewhere, is very much a socially constructed disease, the specific forms of which reflect socio-economic and political conditions over the past several decades. A vocabulary of AIDS has emerged in Uganda reflecting a set of concepts, attitudes and beliefs shared by these social groups while the specific emphasis within each group indicates basic disparities of view.

This chapter is based on eight months's fieldwork in 1991 and forms part of my larger study of the social history and political economy of AIDS in Uganda (British Economic and Social Research Council acknowledgment 1989-1992). In earlier research on the history of sleeping sickness epidemics in colonial Zaire (Lyons 1985, 1988a, 1988b, 1992). I became aware of the wider political, economic, social and cultural issues which form the background to epidemics of disease and responses to them. The intensity and dynamics of the epidemic of HIV/AIDS in Africa can be understood only when it is situated within the broader context of the history of health and medicine, particularly over the past fifty years. Sources of information include government and private archives, the press, religious and non-government organizations, and international and national aid agencies. I collected nearly two hundred interviews in the southern half of the country. While the informants represent many of the national and international agencies involved in health policy and provision as well as practitioners and scientists working directly with HIV/AIDS, the majority were rural dwellers[2]. Questions were designed to probe beyond individual recollections of disease and health management in the past in an effort to elicit deeper attitudes and beliefs concerning the causes of and appropriate responses to illness and misfortune. I was particularly interested in people's attitudes and practices concerning sexuality and sexual disease. Aware of the sensitive nature of my study, I was always careful to introduce myself and to explain the project to local political leaders after which I moved freely[3].

Historically, epidemics have evoked a range of responses from all levels of society and AIDS is no exception. With no cure or vaccine in sight during the first decade of the AIDS epidemic, the world has witnessed a plethora of responses from the purely scientific to accusations of witchcraft and international germ warfare. Clearly, we are experiencing two major epidemics; an epidemic of a deadly virus and an epidemic of signification, or meanings. Language can create an illusion of "reality" in which words seem the transparent medium through which we can "see" the real facts. Critics have suggested that we should attempt to circumvent the "increasingly centralized, professionalized handling of the epidemic" so that "the voices of the third world may lead us to scrutinize the linguistic imperialism that has constructed the very terms . . . AIDS and the Third World" (Treichler 1988:35). I believe, however, that this suggested dichotomy assumes a "reality" in the voices of the Third World masked by first world constructions. While much of the scientific discourse on AIDS in Uganda does indicate the quite different concerns of Ugandan scientists in contrast to those of expatriate, or European scientists, there is a significant degree of interplay in the language which reveals a shared scientific conceptualization of AIDS.

In this chapter I shall explore the language used by a number of social groups in Uganda to discuss AIDS. Beginning with the influential discourse of the experts, the scientists and practitioners, I will then examine the language used in reference to prostitution which is seen by many to be a major factor in the epidemic. Politicians, from the president to local representatives, have been forced to include AIDS on their agendas as have religious leaders and other self-appointed representatives of the moral order. It is not surprising that AIDS, like other sexually transmitted diseases in the past, has evoked a range of emotional responses and in the final section of the chapter I will look at Ugandan discourse on religion, sex and disease.

Medico-Scientific Discourse
and Epidemiological Models

Given the many socio-economic factors which distinguish African populations from those in the West, we have to ask why researchers have chosen to focus on sexual promiscuity in Africa as the major route to understanding the present epidemic of AIDS (Packard 1989)? It is an emphasis which reminds us of centuries-old stereotypes of the "sexually rapacious African" inhabiting a dangerous and diseased continent. From nearly the beginning of scientific research into HIV/AIDS in Uganda, the course was set for the epidemiological explanation. HIV was spread through promiscuous sexuality and Ugandans *are* promiscuous. In the U.S. and Europe there were clearly targeted social groups who engaged in this behavior. In Uganda, it was more problematic but there was widespread consensus by the mid to late 1980s that *Ugandans* are promiscuous. While prostitutes, lorry drivers and businessmen have been targeted for interventions, there remains a widespread assumption that on the whole, African populations consist of highly sexed and sexually active individuals.

The Paradigm

The Ugandan Ministry of Health conducted an early investigation into the strange new disease in Fort Portal in 1985 and reported that "it was agreed it was 'AIDS in the African context'" because in Uganda there are neither homosexuals nor drug abusers (*Weekly Topic*. Kampala, 3 Sup. 1985). Two years later, in 1987, a team of expatriate and Ugandan scientists concluded that in Uganda, "homosexuality and intravenous drug abuse, recognized risk factors in western countries, were not seen as risk factors" (Berkley et al. 1989b).

The problem was to explain why HIV was apparently so widespread in many regions of Africa. Gradually, the scientific community constructed a definition for "African AIDS," distinct from the epidemic in the West. Not everyone agreed. For instance, a black doctor in the United States explained that:

There is a widespread myth that AIDS in Africa, and the way it is transmitted, is somehow different from AIDS in developed countries . . . African AIDS is transmitted in exactly the same way as AIDS in other societies (Duh 1987:53).

A number of important assumptions underpin present ideas of AIDS epidemiology in Africa. The scientific and medical community have constructed a definition of "African AIDS" based on a paradigm which, like all accepted scientific models, has been powerful in its influence and difficult to dislodge.

The dominant paradigm evolved from the early epidemiological analysis of the transmission of HIV in the West where the attention of researchers focussed initially on certain social groups. The major features of this paradigm are:

1. HIV is related to sexual promiscuity and homosexuals are promiscuous.
2. HIV is related to certain "risk behaviors."
3. HIV is related to certain "risk groups," e.g., homosexuals, IV drug users and prostitutes.

This model views the subject as an independent agent with the option of choice. "Risk behavior" implies that the individual has the power of choice and, importantly, it implies responsibility for personal actions. The possibility of infection is very much the choice, therefore the responsibility, of the individual. This paradigm is laden with subjective judgements related to the specific social, economic and political contexts of the West. But when transferred to different cultures and societies, how useful are the terms, "promiscuity," "risk" and "prostitute," which play such an important role in the scientific and medical discourse on AIDS?

In Africa, while the initial paradigm was retained, scientists believed that certain adjustments had to be made in order to explain so-called "African AIDS." HIV seemed more widely dispersed among some populations and was more evenly shared by men and women. How could science explain the heterosexual epidemic in Africa? Thus it was concluded that AIDS in Africa must be different. What is "African AIDS?" The paradigm in Africa was viewed as follows:

1. AIDS in Africa is different from AIDS in the West; in Africa it is an heterosexual, not a homosexual, epidemic (the sex ratio in Africa in the late 1980s was more like 1:1 while in the West it was initially 1 male: 13 female).
2. Africans are promiscuous; African sexuality is a "risk behavior."
3. Risk groups do exist; they include truck drivers, businessmen, bureaucrats, and prostitutes.

Basically, the paradigm retains its major features—promiscuity, prostitutes, risk— with the most significant change being the added adjective, "heterosexual." The onus, however, remains with the individual who is potentially risk-taking and *responsible* for her/his exposure to HIV. This was indeed the major difference in views of the contours of the epidemic in Africa. Left out are the deeper, underlying factors, or the co-factors in epidemiological discourse, of so-called "African AIDS." Nevertheless, the power of the earlier model developed in the United States and Europe maintained a powerful grip on the imaginations of scientists and other researchers in Africa and specific groups—prostitutes, the educated African "elite," and truck drivers—were targeted for intervention strategies in the mid to late 1980s.

Thomas Kuhn has argued that in the history of science, the accepted paradigms, themselves, have acted as powerful constraints to real "leaps" in knowledge, or "breaks" with accepted models. True creativity, deviation from the accepted norm, is difficult and rare:

> No part of the aim of normal science is to call forth new sorts of phenomena; indeed those that will not fit the box are often not seen at all. Nor do scientists normally aim to invent new theories, and they are often intolerant of those invented by others. Instead, normal-scientific research is directed to the articulation of those phenomena and theories that the paradigm supplies (Kuhn 1970).

Much of the social research being conducted in relation to AIDS in Africa continues to remain within the parameters of broader scientific or epidemiological studies designed by "hard" rather than "soft" scientists. Thus, for instance, anthropologists have been employed to test the working hypotheses of scientists concerning African sexuality, promiscuity, risk groups and risk behaviors ("risk group" and "risk behavior" definitions).

A former director of the Ugandan National AIDS Control Programme [ACP] reported in Washington D.C. in 1987 that "transmission of AIDS is propagated by indiscriminate sexual behavior in which high prostitution and promiscuity are important risk factors" (Oware 1987). "Risk group" and "risk behavior" are epidemiological concepts with long histories in relation to sexually transmitted diseases. Risk can be interpreted in two ways with quite important differences of meaning: there are individuals, groups, or even whole countries, "at risk" and, conversely, some individuals or groups engage in "risk behaviors." The first implies "innocence" while the latter implies a degree of responsibility on the part of the people concerned.

Science and Promiscuity. A good example of the discourse of AIDS in "hard science" is that of an influential team at a London University which has been modeling the epidemic using "epidemiological and demographic processes" and whose publications are carefully scrutinized by the international scientific community. Western scientists pay attention to these scientists' views on AIDS in Africa. In 1991 they stated that:

> The higher prevalence of HIV-1 in heterosexual populations in Africa (by comparison with developed countries) has been linked to . . . higher rates of sexual partner change in African societies (Anderson et al. 1991).

Perhaps reflecting a recent sensitivity by scientists in relation to the highly subjective topic of research, African sexuality, these researchers refer to "higher rates of sexual partner change" in place of the ubiquitous "promiscuity" used in much scientific writing. It may be that recent World Health Organization surveys on sexual behavior in Africa which have concluded "somewhat higher rates of sexual partner change than those reported in developed countries, perhaps by a factor of 2" (Anderson 1991) has led to the more restrained language.

In any case, Ugandan scientists, who often take exception to sweeping and unproven generalizations about African behavior and cultures on other occasions, themselves used language which mirrors Western views. In one of the earliest articles about AIDS in their country, Ugandan scientists explained that "a new disease has been recognized in the Rakai district in South West Uganda . . . the syndrome is known locally as slim disease." They added that "it would seem that slim disease is, indeed, recent and that it has spread because of heterosexual promiscuity, which is hard to document in a rural community." It was also noted that "although the subjects in our study deny overt promiscuous behavior, their sexual behavior is, by Western standards, heterosexually promiscuous" (Serwadda et al. 1985). A 1987 article in the *Reviews of Infectious Diseases* reiterated the assertion that "most African societies are promiscuous by Western standards" (Hrdy 1987).

"Western standards" are not described nor are we informed of the methodology of the social survey which resulted in this observation. Two years later, and seven years since AIDS was discussed frankly in Uganda, a group of Western and Ugandan scientists explained that "two common hypotheses to explain high rates of HIV transmission in Africa are promiscuity and high prevalence of co-factors for infection" (Berkeley et al. 1989a:162). They add:

> We demonstrated that most common risk factors for HIV infection in Uganda relate to high-risk heterosexual behavior such as contracting sexually transmitted diseases, having sex with persons with symptomatic HIV infections, and promiscuity (Berkley et al. 1989).

Another "mixed" group of scientists in Uganda qualified "promiscuity" somewhat, with the observation that "numbers of sexual partners was correlated to HIV positivity although correlation was not apparent in males *without* a history of STDs . . . "(Konde-Lule 1989).

Perhaps the most extensive example of the use of the term, "promiscuity" is that in Daniel Hdry's 1987 article in the *Reviews of Infectious Diseases* quoted here at length with omissions:

> . . . promiscuity is correlated not only with matrilineal societies. Many patrilineal African societies are promiscuous as well...transmission of STDs [sexually transmitted diseases] is presumably enhanced by promiscuity . . . the "infertility belt" in areas with a high prevalence of antibody to AIDS virus, which also may be related to promiscuity. As people leave rural villages and migrate to urban areas, the general level of promiscuity usually increases . . . Increased promiscuity is especially common among upper- and middle-class urban men, who can afford the services of prostitutes...levels of STDs are generally high in Africa; this fact may reflect both casual attitudes toward sex and high levels of promiscuity as well as the lack of easily available treatment (Hrdy 1987).

"Promiscuity" is a problematic term in AIDS discourse. It can be argued that scientists use the term objectively since technically, it means "more than one sexual partner." But in Uganda there are a number of readings of "'promiscuous" which all share emotive connotations. How objective is a term which includes among its meanings the notions of "indiscriminate," "haphazard," "casual" or "accidental" in connection with social relations? In fact, I suggest that the term cannot be used scientifically because it implies a notion of "standards," be they ethical, moral, legal, or scientific, to which no society could subscribe in unison.

Scientific Imperialism? Ugandans have expressed some reservations and much anger at the way in which much AIDS research has been dominated by foreign scientists who have quite different motivations. In the earliest days of research in the region [1985], an article in a Kampala weekly newspaper described how in the capital of neighboring Rwanda:

> some doctors are experimenting with suramin on black patients in Kigali . . . strange that Dr. R.C. Gallo found it necessary to reassure the American and European public

saying "we wish to stress the first phase trial is to learn whether the drug can be safely administered to AIDS patients." So they are learning in Africa (*Weekly Topic* 1985).

While the goal of medical research is assumed by most of us to include the discovery of cures and ways to avoid disease, it is significant that Africans give expression to deeply cynical views of the relevance of such medical and scientific research to their own well-being. Prominent Ugandan scientists involved in HIV/AIDS research funded by outside agencies feel that "AIDS researchers in Africa face some difficult problems, several partly self-inflicted or caused by colleagues from overseas." For instance, in their view, the speculation about the African origins of HIV brought an

> influx of scientists trying to prove this theory . . . but early emphasis on "discovering the origin of AIDS in Africa" was pejorative and unfortunate. Many African politicians strongly resented this emphasis, and sensationalized reports in the western mass media had unfortunate results, one of which was that "the motives of foreign researchers were viewed with extreme suspicion."

In addition, continue the Ugandan scientists, there may be:

> a divergence between the goals of African and of western researchers . . . it sometimes seems that researchers (and funding agencies) from overseas find it easier than their local colleagues to overlook the suffering caused by AIDS to individuals and communities in Africa (Serwadda et al. 1990).

They concluded with a plea for greater financial commitment to the clinical needs of the study population, and towards training of local experts. There have been enough sero-surveys, head counts of HIV infected individuals, complains an African physician. What is needed now, is not more seroepidemiology, but some clinical epidemiology. The administrator of Nsambya Hospital in Kampala, considered by many to be the best equipped and most fully functioning hospital in Uganda is:

> saddened by the way external research agencies lost interest whenever she mentioned the need for strengthening her clinical epidemiological research base to enable her go round the villages to follow up and treat patients with AIDS...Research funds must never be for service ("that is the sole burden of the Ugandan government"), she seems to have been told, but are for taking the blood of as many people as possible to measure "seropositivity" and T lymphocytes. A field unit in south western Uganda does not have to rely on seroepidemiology to gauge the spread and seriousness of AIDS in Africa (Konotey-Ahulu 1987:1593-94).

A rather stunning example of the real difference in interests of Ugandan and western scientists was revealed dramatically at a recent public meeting convened in Kampala by World Health Organization officials on the subject of possible vaccine trials in the country. In the presence of more than 200 people who attended, the director of the newly formed Ugandan National AIDS Commission and chair of the meeting, asked the WHO officials, "are we going to be used as guinea pigs or play an important role in the development of a vaccine?" An evocative metaphor, *guinea pig,* was used in this context to refer to the neo-colonial relations of Western and African science. Additionally, there was reference to the larger race and class issues. Other members of the Ugandan audience queried how the illiterate peasantry could be adequately informed about the research in order to give "informed consent." The World Health Official representative responded by explaining that,"illiteracy does not mean that a person is not clever."

Expressing a widely-held view in Uganda that HIV had been introduced into Africa by the World Health Organization during the smallpox eradication campaign in the 1970s, another member of the audience asked, "how can we be sure that this vaccine won't come here and finish the job?" His question, with its hint of a gangland "hit man," elicited an emotional response from the World Health Organization representative. The answer revealed deep misunderstanding on the part of the foreigners and their lack of knowledge of the discourse of AIDS inside Uganda: "If there are such suspicions, Uganda might not be a good testing site. He added, however, that any vaccine which might result from testing in a developing country would be "economically appropriate," adding "We will not develop a Rolls Royce vaccine here" (Zarembo 1991).

The Woman on the Street. President Museveni asserted in November 1990 that "the main route of AIDS is through prostitution" (New Vision, November 15, 1990). As mentioned earlier, while *Africans* in general are labeled "promiscuous" by scientists and others, there has been much emphasis on specific sub-groups such as prostitutes, businessmen and lorry drivers. In 1985, in a seminal article describing "Slim, a new disease in Uganda," Ugandan scientists concurred that, "prostitutes and traveling traders are potential sources of infection" (Serwadda et al. 1985).

Most scientific and medical references to "prostitutes" in Uganda are made without explanation or terms of reference, it being assumed that the reader possesses a clear definition of "prostitute" as well as a knowledge of the forms of sexual exchange pertaining to persons of different cultures and societies in that country. Women are beginning to react to simplistic labeling. One woman, for instance, recently discussed how "all Ugandan women who go to Dubai have been labelled as dirty, loose, indecent . . . in other words, prostitutes." Dubai is an important trading center for many Ugandan business people. Women who have been able to afford to build their own houses have been included within the rubric of prostitute. In the writer's view:

> history has proved that wherever women seek economic independence they are castigated for prostituting...I remember that the first women who disentangled themselves from customary constraints and went to "Buganda" . . . to work for money were all labelled as delinquents and prostitutes (Bagyendera 1991).

Nonetheless, the labelling continues. A 1988 study of HIV/AIDS in two rural mission hospitals in southwestern Uganda by a team of scientists from Cambridge University concluded that "AIDS in Africa appears to be primarily spread by sexual contact between men and prostitutes . . . "

Who were the prostitutes? We are told that "a cohort of thirty-six suspected prostitutes" was compared to another of thirty-six "married women." Lacking a more precise methodology, the Cambridge researchers simply labelled as prostitutes those women who, formerly married, were *apparently* without men at the time of the study (Hudson et al. 1988).

Influential persons frequently point to prostitutes as a potentially dangerous and polluting group which poses a threat to the wider society. A former director of the AIDS Control Programme explained that "when you touch a prostitute you have touched the disease. Be careful and protect yourselves." Referring to individual responsibility, he continued, "AIDS is the only disease where you can choose to have it or not" (*New Vision*, July 13, 1990).

Numbers of local political leaders have publicly condemned prostitution and made a plea for concerned citizens to suggest ways to stamp it out (Owor 1990). In one district it was decided that:

> any person who practices prostitution commits an offence and on conviction must be sentenced to six months imprisonment after which, she must be deported to her local area of origin (*New Vision*, December 14, 1990).

It must be conceded that HIV is widely transmitted in Uganda as an STD but we need to remember that like all STDs there are certain predisposing co-factors in the successful transmission of the virus. By late 1990, this had become increasingly clear as scientists discerned the relationship between HIV transmission and the presence of sexually transmitted diseases, especially those genital urinary diseases accompanied by ulceration which allows more successful penetration of HIV. Dr. Richard Goodgame who spent some years in Uganda discussed the importance of co-factors:

> Studies have shown an association of HIV infection in Africa with increased numbers of sexual partners (five refs), a history of sexually transmitted disease or genital ulcers, the presence of an intact foreskin . . .

Nevertheless, he stressed the importance of "a history of prostitution or sexual contact with a prostitute," and explained that, "high risk groups do exist. In Uganda, barmaids and truck drivers, for instance." Unlike most epidemiological accounts in Uganda which I have seen, Goodgame added the qualification that once seroprevalence surpasses 10%, "the usefulness of risk-group identification in patient care begins to diminish" (Goodgame 1990). Some men are taking no chances at all, thus avoiding the need to identify dangerous sub-groups. A local political representative explained to me that "we suspect that every woman has AIDS...that is how one can keep out of danger . . ." More direct action is taken in some areas like Rakai District in 1986 where it was reported that:

> teenage girls and young women in their thirties are being arrested and deported from the area for fear they could be AIDS carriers. This is especially true in the case of girls new to the area (*Weekly Topic*, March 1986).

Politicians and AIDS

The politics of health are very much on the agenda in many parts of the world and the role of the state in relation to the health of its population is a contentious issue. In Uganda where AIDS has been described as "cataclysmic" and "potentially devastating," no politician can afford to ignore the issue. Museveni pointed out the sheer political necessity of paying attention to AIDS by reminding local political leaders at a meeting that "politicians derive their strength from people and so need to protect their constituencies." Museveni went on to explain that "since 1981 AIDS had assumed alarming proportions and [he] blamed past governments for failing to tackle the problem (Bitangaro 1991). In December 1985, a letter from a concerned citizen had asked "what is the government doing? [AIDS] is not even mentioned by Government officials" (Mulwindwa 1990).

With the advent of the NRM Government of Yoweri Museveni in February 1986, this was to change and Uganda became one of the earliest countries in Sub-Saharan Africa to welcome discourse and research on AIDS within its borders. But the nature of that "openness" can be qualified through examination of the content of some AIDS discourse. We have already seen how political leaders, including the president, added their voices to the ground swell of opinion that prostitutes must be "stamped out." Unfortunately, much of the language used by Ugandan political leaders in reference to AIDS was filled with rhetorical moralistic messages.

It is interesting how Museveni's discussion of AIDS in relation to African "tradition" has altered over time. In December 1990 Museveni lashed out at the "traditions and customary habits, like polygamous marital relations which encouraged the spread of the killer disease...[and said that there was need to revise] some of our laws which encourage immorality and promiscuity..." (Museveni 1990).

Six months later, in his speech at the 7th International Conference on AIDS in Florence on 16th June 1991, Museveni explained that "young people must be taught the virtues of abstinence, self-control and postponement of pleasure and sometimes, sacrifice" (International Conference on AIDS 1991). But in the same speech and much to the consternation of those in the audience awaiting a clear declaration of approval of condom usage from the President of Uganda, Museveni added that in the past

> to discourage the spread of these diseases [STDs] in society, Africans had evolved cultural taboos against premarital sex and strict sanctions had been established against premarital sex or sex out of wedlock.

And he said that he has been:

> emphasizing a return to our time tested cultural practices which emphasized fidelity and condemnation of pre-marital or extra-marital sex. I believe that the best response to the threat posed by AIDS and other sexuality transmitted diseases is to reaffirm publicly and forthrightly the reverence and respect and responsibility every person owes his or her neighbor (*New Vision* 1991).

Moving from his attack on "African tradition" made only six months earlier, the president now referred to cultural traditions, especially those of the mythical, golden age variety, in the hope of effecting behavioral change.

A mere two months later, August 1991, at a seminar on AIDS for National Resistance Council members, the Ugandan president turned to the subject of "foreign cultures," which he accused of helping "in the spread of AIDS." To illustrate, he called for an end to the practice of "boyfriend / girlfriend," adding that for people close to him, he had banished the "boyfriend/ girlfriend business." He said, "Dating? What is dating? Why don't they talk here in front of me?." And returning to the discourse on traditional values, he explained, "in the past, we had tribal cultures which were very complete although somehow conservative. But what have you put in its place?" Curiously, Museveni believes that "in the past...traditional medicine was associated with evil but it was up to leaders [now] to help the public change their attitude about it."

At every political level, politicians have been responding to the fears of their constituencies. In Rakai District, for example, pressured by a number of women's groups, political leaders have decided to avoid the spread of AIDS by banning discos in schools while discos and wedding parties, traditionally occasions of much sexual adventure, should take place during the day. Furthermore, it was suggested that "treatment of hair of any kind and wearing of ear-rings should be prohibited" (Kalibbala 1991).

Coffins or Condoms?:
The Great Moral Debate (New Vision 1991)

AIDS discourse attains hysterical proportion on the subject of condoms. It is perhaps the condom which has occasioned the most heated debate involving as it does a range of issues important in the African context. These include population control, the power to control one's own sexuality, and deeply entrenched religious objections. The condom issue involves all strata of society and Ugandan politicians, religious leaders and citizens discuss a wide range of social, economic and political issues. Attitudes range from "condoms are not African," "condoms will promote promiscuity and moral lassitude," "condoms are a ploy to control our population size," "condoms kill women," "condoms are evil" to "condoms will hinder the reconstruction of Uganda."

With no cure or vaccine for AIDS in sight the principle public health message worldwide has been "use condoms." But in many lesser developed countries where the subject of population control is politically sensitive, efforts to introduce family planning ideologies and methods in past decades have encountered much resistance. Some have complained that such campaigns are motivated by a "western plot" to control third world populations. Alternatively, religious leaders warn that attempts to limit family size are "against nature," evil and sinful.

AIDS, as a sexually transmitted disease, has forced proponents for and against contraception into open confrontations to the extent that in Uganda recently, there was a call for parliamentary debate on the issue of the morality of public health programs which propound the use of condoms to save lives. In 1991 Uganda's bishops condemned a health policy which advises people to use condoms. The church leaders were not without opposition, however. One man suggested that the Bishops "follow court processes to obtain judicial ruling on the matter if they can prove any substantial damage done to them personally or to their interests" (Amati-Aiah 1991).

A strongly worded editorial entitled, "Churchmen: give the condom a chance" made clear that all Ugandans are faced with "a simple matter of opportunity cost; a choice between a sure coffin and a condom that reduces the chances of death." Appealing to a rather different sense of responsibility, the editorial continued that it is:

> therefore shocking that top leadership of Catholic and Protestant churches over the weekend came out strongly against the use of condoms, on grounds that the small innocent rubber will spread immorality . . . this is not the time to engage in academic and moralistic debates when human lives are at stake. What the churchmen should tell us is why their opposition to condoms comes now when about 2 million people are infected. They should tell us how their 'morality;' which couldn't check AIDS in the mid-eighties will do miracles now in the nineties...let the Ministry of Health do its practical duty and save those who can't be saved by morality as you see it....until a cure is found the catch word shall be: ABSTAIN, BUT IF YOU CANNOT, THEN PROTECT OR PERISH (*Weekly Topic* 1991).

A Ugandan physician acting as AIDS Coordinator in Fort Portal explained that:

> using a condom is like taking chloroquine tablets. They are bitter, have some side effects, have a terrible taste but if you live in an area full of malaria and you are not immune, you must take chloroquine as a prophylactic . . . the "bitter pill" for prevention. The condom is the same (Bitaroho-Kabwa 1991).

In contrast to its early, open policy vis-a-vis the international scientific community and HIV/AIDS research within its boundaries, Ugandan leaders and scientists have been reluctant to confront directly the difficult issue of condoms. In 1989 the head of the ACP warned that:

We have to be cautious about advocating condom use until we fully understand local cultural practices and attitudes. The Ugandan AIDS education campaign is not centered on the promotion of use of prophylactics as similar programs in the US and Europe (Berkly 1989).

In 1991 the director of the ACP reiterated the very qualified recommendation on condoms saying that 'they should not replace morality and discipline'. And enlisting a much-used rationalization, he explained that, after all

Condoms are 90 percent effective in family planning as a contraceptive and not 100 percent in preventing AIDS. He therefore said they [the ACP] do not advocate for condoms as a principle, but only in limited circumstances (Berkly et al. 1989b).

An AIDS counselor at a prominent mission hospital referred to his dilemma as a health worker and a Catholic:

In fact, from the religious point of view, the condom is not recommended but from the medical point of view it is recommendable. It leaves us in a big puzzle. We display the cards to the patient and tell him the good and evil of using it.

When asked, "What is the evil in using a condom?" he explained that "God doesn't allow it, it is not good. From a medical point of view it is not 100% safe. I have not seen any condoms at Kitovu (Kazibwe 1991)." In another mission hospital a Ugandan medical assistant told me that they "tend to avoid propounding the use of condoms because it isn't really 100%." Instead, he said they "strongly advise a man to stay with the woman God has brought you together with...try to avoid temptations" (Enyodo interview 1990).

The specious argument that condoms are not 100% effective for either contraception or prophylaxis is employed by spokesmen for both science and religion. Another strand of this argument concerns the quality of condoms sent to Uganda. Many believe that condoms supplied by USAID, for example, have exceeded their shelf-life. While there may be some degree of truth in this observation, such reasoning can be confused with untruths which may seriously impede public health efforts. Consider the words of this woman in Kabale District who explained that

a woman told us about a condom in All Saints Church when she was teaching us about slim. She told us that a condom is worn by a man for sexual intercourse to avoid sexual diseases. She told us that a condom is dangerous. They spend a long time on the way and by the time they are brought this way, they are old. So if a man uses it, it breaks and kills a woman (Kyarisiima interview 1990).

One of the very few AIDS counselors in a very large region of the southwest of Uganda explained how he, like the young man cited above, resolved the contradiction posed by condoms for the religious health worker:

> We as a church do not approve the use of condoms. We have a commandment which God put there: never commit adultery. That's that, finished. If we allowed use of condoms as a church we would be encouraging sexual immorality and if you die because of a sexual immorality you will perish (Katonbozi interview 1990).

There is clearly an important distinction between a "mere" death caused by AIDS and perishing in the sense of infinite banishment from God's grace. Given the choice, according to the religious discourse, one would prefer to die a moral death. This point was considered by a recent editorial which suggested that "many of the Ugandan priests who have died of AIDS or committed suicide as a result would still be alive if they had not preferred 'live moral sex' to the 'protected immoral one'" (*Weekly Topic* 1991).

Religion, Sex, and Disease: "Evil, be thou my good"

Like their counterparts elsewhere Ugandan religious leaders have responded vehemently to public health campaigns propounding the prophylactic use of condoms. And in common with a great many non-Western, lesser developed countries suffering widespread poverty and lack of education, Uganda contains a highly vocal and extensive network of religious leaders. Catholics, Protestants, Traditionalists, Muslims and ever increasing numbers of fundamentalist, "born-again" Christians have been a potent source of opinion and influence in relation to AIDS and to all public health efforts to contain the epidemic, claiming that "AIDS is God-sent and this is because people sinned and God sent a plague as punishment. We shall all die one day" (*New Vision* 1990). People explain that there is "no cure which is a sign of punishment" (*New Vision* 1987).

The confusion of morality with public health is increased by sensitivities related to religious affiliation. A Muslim complained about the religious bias of a major newspaper in Kampala which published the following advertisement: The Bible may save your soul but this condom will save your life. He complained that

> the constant reference to the Bible makes the caption lop-sided and biased as the word Bible has little meaning to our Moslem brothers. I suggest therefore that as your readership is not entirely Christian, you alternate the word "Bible" with "Koran" to allow your anti-aids caption to give some more meaning to our Moslem brothers. Until then you are practicing sectarianism (Kasangati 1991).

Traditional religious leaders, like this Muganda *nabbi*, or prophet-healer in Rakai District, have their own explanations. Linking AIDS with the wider cultural and political process of the Baganda, he said that

> AIDS is a method God has used to turn back the clock to our traditional laws . . . it is now a hundred years since people turned away from God...AIDS will disappear when we [the Baganda] have the Kabaka back (Nabbi interview 1991).

The kabaka was the traditional ruler, or king, of the Baganda, the large and influential ethnic group favored by the British administration throughout the colonial period. Exiled by the British in 1953, the kabaka was still, in 1991, missed by many Baganda who viewed him as a unifying factor in their culture. In this example, the looming apocalypse so often forecast in reference to AIDS in Uganda was seen as intimately related to the disturbed state of political relations among one of the major populations of Uganda. AIDS is "the curse of the Kabaka." The *nabbi* continued his explanation:

> AIDS can be cured but we have to go back to our culture . . . When people have sexual intercourse, they use the whites' way of kissing the private parts, this causes God's wrath, God will punish the people who started this habit...Anyone who does not regain his cultural values will surely die as I tell my people every day (Nabbi interview 1991).

Some religious leaders have found the AIDS epidemic to be an opportunity to garner souls. A mission doctor explained that the major risk factor for AIDS is promiscuity and that polygamy, widely practiced in his region, is a "form of promiscuity." When asked what he could do to help Ugandans, he said "Really the only help is our Christian message which can empower a person to live morally...we believe this is the only help." Turning his attention to people who already have AIDS, he said he was pleased

> if they find meaning, values and a sense of dignity through AIDS . . . it really heartens us when we see people really saved when they know they are terminal. As Christians we feel the only answer to AIDS is Christianity (Dr. I.S. interview 1990).

Conclusion

In this paper I have discussed several issues which have emerged in the discourse on AIDS in Uganda ranging from the "official" scientific perceptions to those of the common citizen. In Uganda, we can see an "epidemic of signification" and the creation of particular sub-cultures. Scientific discourse is of prostitutes, lorry drivers and businessmen while ordinary citizens include "Dubai traders," foreigners and women. At times of epidemic sexually transmitted diseases, "pathological others" are created partly as explanation and partly to avoid moral stigma. A problem arises, however, with the confusion of the concepts of "risk behavior," "people at risk" and "pathological others." Epidemiological categories are confused with moral precepts which can hinder public health policy.

Notes

1.   The interviews on which this study is based were carried out at Makerere University, Kampala in August 1988. Several interviews were also conducted with members of the National AIDS Control Program and at Mulago Hospital. Funds for this research were provided by the HIV Center for Clinical and Behavioral Studies at Columbia University.

2.   Ugandan anthropologist, Christine Obbo, has begun to trace AIDS deaths among small clusters within such networks and to explore High School students' attitudes toward "elite deaths" (1991).

3.   It must be stressed that these were *reported* AIDS cases. Of these, 90% had serum drawn for testing and were sero-positive for HIV-1 antibodies by ELISA. Other cases were reported on the basis of the Uganda clinical case definition for AIDS. Social and behavioral attributes of AIDS cases were not routinely recorded and the data appears to be collected for clinical rather than behavioral analysis. Of the 96% of the cases for which gender was recorded, 47% were male and 53% female. Mean age for males was 28.7 years and for females 24.6 years. Of the 49% for which residence was reported, 46% were urban and 54% rural.

PART THREE

Policy Issues

10

The HIV Epidemic as a Development Issue

Elizabeth Reid

Introduction:
Conceptual Complexity

There are two important characteristics of the HIV epidemic which need to be acknowledged and understood, by national leaders in particular, for they will affect and determine the nature of the response to the epidemic in the Asian and Pacific region.

First, the epidemic is at one and the same time both a crisis and an endemic condition. It is a crisis because the speed of spread of this virus can be so awesome. Infection rates can, and have even in this region, increased from two per cent to 25 per cent in adult populations in less than four years. There is no reason to assume that this is not happening in this region. Before people are even aware that they are surrounded by infected family and friends, their communities have been deeply penetrated. This fact alone should be sufficient for the epidemic to be viewed as a calamity, albeit too often invisible in its early stages, as much in need of an immediate response as the invasion of one country by another. For war nowadays rarely has the toll in human lives that this virus is causing and will cause.

That it is an endemic condition may best be simply illustrated by the fact that, even if in an affected country there were to be no further cases of infection as from today, the pain and trauma of the deaths of those already infected will continue for the next twenty years and the social and economic repercussions of their deaths will continue on for decades and generations after that. We know that nowhere in the world is the spread abating or even slowing down. Each day of continuing spread adds to the ramifications and duration of its devastating impact. Both dimensions, the epidemic as crisis and the epidemic as endemic, need to be recognized. Each has its own appropriate responses.

Second, the epidemic manifests itself both as a specific problem but also as a pervasive one. Its specificity is revealed in its associated morbidity and mortality, in increasing numbers of people, mostly healthy, productive young women and men, getting sick and dying. The response of the first decade of the epidemic addressed this quality of the epidemic. It focused on the epidemic as a health crisis and on its ramifications for health service delivery.

However, the repercussions of these deaths will permeate and affect every facet of human life and national development, more so in countries where men and women are infected in more or less the same numbers. The causes and the consequences of the spread of the virus embrace poverty and wealth, disempowerment and influence, well-being and disease, deprivation and development, trust and bad faith; the very way we are as human beings.

Both of these dimensions of the epidemic, its particularity and its ubiquity, must also be recognized. Each of these too has its own appropriate responses. Thus this epidemic is conceptually complex: at once a crisis and an endemic condition; at once a specific issue and a permeating one.

Program Imperatives

These two characteristics of the HIV epidemic impose a set of imperatives upon us:

1. The imperative of an effective response.
2. The imperative of a sustainable response.
3. The imperative of a coordinated response.

The prerequisite of an effective response is a common understanding of the nature of the epidemic, which takes into account the above two characteristics, and a shared vision of the way forward. This we do not yet have. This should not surprise us for the epidemic is a new and complex phenomenon for which there is no likeness in living memory, not one drawn from war, not from disease, not from natural disasters, nor from man-made ones.

This is not to say that we are blindly groping. We are doing what we know needs to be done while we search for new and more effective ways to respond. The more we share a vision of an effective way forward, the more coordination and the building of partnerships will naturally follow.

The second imperative is that of a sustainable response. The commitment and contributions of affected individuals and communities have yet to be recognized or valued but they are extensive. They lie at the heart of a sustainable response to this epidemic but in most cases they need to be supplemented by further human and financial resources. The closeness of these individuals and communities to the problems and needs created by the epidemic generally ensures that their responses are appropriate. Similarly, governments are increasingly beginning to allocate national resources to the epidemic although in most cases they still have to be persuaded that it affects all aspects of societal development both now and in the future.The required human and financial resources must be available for effective responses. However, these responses must also be ranked in order of effectiveness since resources, whether of individuals, communities, nations or of external support agencies, will continue to be limited and will themselves be reduced by the epidemic.

Thus priority must be given to strengthening national capacity to ensure that these resources, and that of the external support agencies, are used in the most effective manner. There is not time and there are not sufficient resources for ill-conceived, inappropriate or ineffective responses. The selection must be ruthless for the demand on resources, both human and financial, will continue and increase inexorably for decades. Communities and governments must have the ability to monitor, assess and evaluate their interventions and to modify, redesign and expand them. Where the response to the epidemic is effective and sustainable, hope is brought into being that the desolation and distress of this epidemic can be eased, a hope that can turn back the tides of fatalism and despair.

The third imperative, that of a coordinated response, means that we must build the partnerships required to ensure that the search for effective and sustainable policies and interventions is an ongoing process and that duplication is minimized. Such partnerships are needed among the community groups responding to the epidemic, between such groups and government, among government ministries, between the public and the private sectors, among external support agencies, especially within the UN system, and between donors and countries.

The Challenges to be Shared

Before we elaborate further on the partnerships required by this epidemic, we need to identify the challenges facing the Asian and Pacific region that we are being called upon to share. I want to identify just three such challenges:

1. The challenge of making the invisible visible.
2. The challenge of creating an ethic of compassion.
3. The challenge of placing people and their communities at the center of the response to the epidemic.

The first challenge, to make the invisible visible, is a clear imperative in this region. We must find the means to better understand and make known the speed and the surreptitious patterns of spread of the virus. Surveillance systems tell us where the virus has been but we need predictive systems that map out for us where it is likely to go. Understanding the factors which determine this will enable us to put faces to the figures, to see ourselves in its path or in its wake.

But more than just numbers and silhouettes of those affected need to be made visible. Those living within the epidemic, those at the forefront of change, must create a new language that makes more visible the new realities of life in the post-HIV era.

This is already happening in two important aspects of the epidemic. Firstly, we are beginning to develop a language of optimism: affirmations of the possibility of behavior change, of the centrality of compassion and concern, of care and commitment. Secondly, we are developing a language of process rather than of interventions, of people as responsible actors rather than manipulable objects. It is a language of empowerment, of participation, of listening and talking, of counseling, of deciding together.

However, there is still a silence, an inarticulateness, about the dark side of the epidemic: the doubt, the trembling, the uncertainty, the distancing, the denial, the fear. We do not yet have a language that reflects the reality of living with the knowledge that one is infected or that someone one loves dearly is infected: the constant companion of mortality, the sadness, the tentativeness of desire, the longing for love, the stripping raw of self by death after death after death of partners, of children, of childhood friends, of companions.

There is another silence around a central reality of this epidemic: that it evokes a wilderness of emotional and psychological states with whose very existence we are uncomfortable, for which our vocabulary is too limited and which we are reluctant to acknowledge and express. These include hatred, anger, shame, guilt, humiliation, grief, indignity. There is a deep unease which permeates families and societies about using a language of sexuality, of mortality and of vulnerability.

Even those emotional states we value and which are central to our belief that the epidemic can be overcome, we hesitate publicly to acknowledge and express. We lack a familiarity of usage of words such as care, compassion, happiness, humility and wonder. For that which is invisible about this epidemic to be made visible, we must spin this language, weave it into our lives and grow strong in the courage to use it.

The second challenge we face is to create an ethic of compassion. Let me begin by delineating what this is not. Compassion is not pity, which strips one of dignity and individuality. Compassion cannot be expressed in authoritarian relationships structurally based on inequalities of power: doctor and patient, men and women, parent and child, caste and class. For this reason an ethics of compassion will threaten conventions of distancing and objectivity, norms of control and domination, prerogatives of position and wealth.

An ethic of compassion will value concern over ambition, connectedness over individualism, closeness over control, mercy over judgement. An ethic of compassion will require the presence of men who pay attention to daily life.

An ethic of compassion is not a matter of appeasing hunger, of providing shelter, of resolving conflict. These are as compatible with charity or pragmatism as with compassion. Rather it involves seeing ourselves as one with others, our lives essentially intertwined with their lives.

An ethic of compassion will bring a particular focus to our work. It will add a sense of urgency to keeping people uninfected. It will place high importance on keeping those affected by the epidemic, the infected, those who love and care for them and those who survive them, within our families, workplace and communities.

Keeping those infected alive for as long as possible will be not only an economic imperative but also a human imperative for even when sick and dying, those infected can nurture their children, touching them, smiling, talking, keeping them company, and can pass on to them their own skills for economic survival, be they farming, brewing, fishing, street selling, cobbling, weaving, repairing or whatever.

Helping those infected to die with dignity through, for example, the treatment of opportunistic infections or the provision of shelter and assistance, will reduce the psychological trauma of the children left behind. Their memories will be of the person they loved not of their unseemly condition.

The third challenge is that of placing people and their communities at the center of the response to the epidemic. Again this can be defined by contrast. It means that primary focus will not be placed on technologies (condoms, test kits, etc.) or on interventions (education campaigns, STD services, for example) but on the initiation of processes whereby both individuals and communities can change and through which agents of change are created. The technologies and interventions will become the handmaidens of, not the masters of, change, there to be called upon as required.

Placing people at the center of the response to the epidemic will enable that response to reflect and build upon the complex nature of people's daily lives and to address their needs in a cohesive manner. It will begin the process of breaking down a compartmentalized development approach to essentially interlinked conditions: poverty, disempowerment, disease, subordination, illiteracy, land ownership, to mention a few, and HIV infection. It recognizes and accepts that little is simple in the face of this epidemic.

An approach that values and builds on the vagaries of human life and human nature will lead to realistic and therefore sustainable responses. It will provide the basis for the hope, the belief, that we are not powerless in the face of this pathogen and that we will indeed overcome the epidemic and its consequences.

The most striking feature about this epidemic is that individuals and communities have been mobilized and empowered by it. People are speaking out; community groups are coming into existence. We see this already in this region. There are many men and women in our communities, speaking out, working with others. However, in a non-supportive environment, too often the impact of such individual initiatives wanes over time as people move on or die or groups lose their initial momentum.

The Partnerships to be Built

The energy, vision and commitment of these agents of change needs to be transformed into an active force for change, a force which can transcend the particular and permeate communities and nations. For this to happen, four social contracts or partnerships must be built.

The first partnership must be a new social contract between men and women. The HIV epidemic and its impact will only be overcome if men and women begin to forge true partnerships of mutual respect and trust and of equitable sharing of the burdens of sadness, pain, care and support created by the epidemic. Men and women must seek to establish the kind of honest communication about sexuality and sexual behavior needed to prevent the transmission of HIV in their partnerships. They must work to restructure the sexual relationships in which they take part.

Women alone cannot stop this epidemic nor care for its sick and its survivors. Women alone cannot bear the burden of its psychological, social and economic impact. Nor should this be expected of them. To do so would be to build in the certainty of failure. Not because of any failing in women, but because sexuality, love and coping are essentially shared experiences.

Changes in individual relationships between men and women will occur only in the context of the emergence of a new social contract, not one simply governing men's or women's behavior, but one which changes what it is to be a man or a women. The social contract must encompass the way we nurture and raise our children, the way society constructs its gender archetypes. It must further allow for community explorations of the appropriateness of accepted community values and standards of behavior. Such a social contract must be supported and reaffirmed by laws, policy, budgetary priorities and program design and delivery.

The family in all its diverse forms thus becomes the basic nexus of change. For although individual men and women can decide on ways to protect themselves from infection, the likelihood of this happening and being sustained resides in factors which long precede adulthood and sexual activity. They have their origin in how people are brought up in family life, whether that be an extended or nuclear family or another environment.

It is in the family context, from birth, that personalities are formed, gender identity is created, moral values are instilled. In particular, it is in families that boys are brought up to be boys, and girls, girls, with their attendant sexual and social identities, attitudes and behaviors. We know that self respect, self confidence, respect for others and an ability to talk about personal and intimate matters are all characteristics which help people to remain uninfected.

Thus it is within family contexts that the basic prevention strategies must be put into place. Love and nurturing must be given to both boys and girls so that they may grow into independent, confident human beings, able to form respectful and non-violent relationships, whatever their sexual orientation may be. Parental-child discourse must be developed on bodily care and sexuality and strengthened on community norms and moral values, especially with regard to respect for self and others. We must change the ways that girls and boys are raised so that as adults they will be less likely to put themselves and others at risk of infection. This will require significant changes in the social construction of masculinity and femininity.

These gender paradigms must be reconstructed in particular ways. The new paradigms should lead to the greater valuing of compassion, concern for others and love of family in men and, for women, in a simple recognition of their value and worth. It is hard to reconcile the oft claimed valuing of women, even as mothers, with the widespread acceptance of female infanticide or the mortality rates associated with pregnancy and childbirth, as high as one woman in 21 in some parts of the world: 1 million women per year. New patterns for the sharing of the responsibilities and joys of women's lives must emerge.

But families individually do not determine cultural meanings, social customs or community values. They inherit, accept, respect and instil them. Thus, for families to change, communities and societies must also change. The new social contract will therefore require a radical reassessment by societies of the very way men and women see themselves and each other, of the way they relate as husband and wife, lovers, brothers and sisters, parent and child, as partners, colleagues and friends.

The second partnership must be a social contract between the affected and the not yet directly affected. The infected and those close to them are amongst the most powerful agents of change in the world today. They can give us glimpses of how we can peacefully co-exist with the virus, of how we can become empowered through the trauma and the tragedy of the epidemic. Within the desolation of this epidemic, they give us snatches of laughter and happiness. They can help us explore and better understand the nature of intimacy, desire and sexuality in the age of the virus.

But these insights of the affected will not be shared, this gift will remain ungiven, if, in the sharing, the affected are stripped of their self esteem and dignity, subjected to humiliation and discrimination, left alone in a hostile limelight without support and companionship. These insights, these glimpses of the world within the epidemic, must be shared if our response is to be grounded in human experience, if this experience and knowledge is to shape and reshape theory and practice.

The stories of the affected provide access to lives which are subtle and various, which present the experience of living within the epidemic in the complex, interrelated way life usually asserts itself. The stories bring to light different perspectives, different points of view and so make the understanding of how to live with the epidemic accessible across class, gender, educational and lifestyle barriers.

Women are more aware of the dynamics of gender in their daily lives. Thus how gender affects the epidemic emerges more clearly in their stories. Life situations such as being infected or caring for someone infected can be understood only if gender roles and interrelationships are taken into account. Women's stories both present and interpret the dynamics of power between women and men and the relationship between the individual and society. They provide glimpses into men's lives as well as into women's lives and relate individual agency to social and economic structures.

Stories, however, do not capture systems of relationships which affect individuals but whose locus is beyond the individual and her or his realm of vision. The relationships between poverty and infection status may form a critical part of the story but the relationships between structural adjustment programs, for example, and poverty, and the tragedy of being infected may not. Hence, stories need to be complemented by system level analyses. A full understanding of the nature and impact of the epidemic requires both kinds of analysis.

This partnership between the affected and their communities is critical. It is an acknowledgment within the community that the epidemic concerns the community as a whole and not just certain individuals perceived or assumed to be at risk. The absence of this social contract favors discrimination, marginalization, denial and infection. The Them/Us mentality which dominates in the absence of this partnership has, sadly, too often characterized perceptions of and responses to the epidemic. There is no Other in the shadow of the epidemic. We are all there.

This second partnership or social contract, once in place, will enable the creation of a supportive milieu that encourages the affected to speak out, tell their stories, reflect on their lives and hopes and help us all to live peacefully with this epidemic.

The third social contract must be between communities and government. The responses we have seen occurring within affected communities provide us with the hope that the epidemic can be overcome, and the insights into how this can come about. These responses are universal. Wherever the virus has spread, communities have responded, to provide care and support, to stop further infection, to assure the rights of the affected, to minister to spiritual, emotional and physical needs.

But individuals, families and communities cannot carry this epidemic alone. There must be a social contract, a partnership, between governments and affected communities. Governments must provide an enabling environment that will evoke, nourish and sustain these responses. This enabling environment must include national policies that acknowledge the centrality of community responses, a body of legal and human rights laws that respect the principles of non-discrimination and respect for the rights and dignity of affected individuals, mechanisms for interaction between government and communities, and assistance, as required, for program design, delivery and financing by communities.

The need for additional resources for this epidemic is frequently mentioned. Whilst it is clear that external resources are needed, it is important to stress that the initial financial resources mobilized to respond to this epidemic are invariably those of individuals, families and communities. As yet, these remain unrecognized and unquantified. We must name these contributions and quantify them for, sadly, this is the way that most people recognize and establish the value of such actions.

These resources—peoples' volunteered time, the food, means and insights they share, the transport provided, the labor contributed, the funds raised—lie at the heart of a sustainable response.

Yes, the resources must be supplemented. They are not without end. They themselves are depleted by the epidemic. They are not, always or usually, sufficient. Communities know what additional resources, human or financial, they need for sustenance and growth. They need to be empowered to be able to define their external support requirements, select them, manage them and account for them in appropriate ways whether these resources come from national or international sources. Mutual trust and respect is a *sine qua non* for a social contract between communities and their government. This may not be easy for either but it must come about.

The fourth partnership must be a global contract. As the epidemic deepens, its devastating potential impact on all aspects of human life and national development is becoming better understood. Certain nations may be brought towards the threshold of destitution. Will the world wait until this stage is reached in some countries? When will there be a global response? Will the world community provide the resources for investment in the education, health and social welfare of people and in the technological development required to enable these nations to continue to function? Will there be global social safety nets to allow nations rendered poor by this epidemic, and the poor within nations, to survive?

The working of global trade agreements and markets have increased the disparities between rich and poor nations and rich and poor individuals. At the national level, many governments try to offset such tendencies by redistributing income through systems of progressive income tax and by supplementing this with social safety nets to prevent people from falling into poverty and absolute destitution. No such systems exist at present at the global level.

The closest the world comes to a global safety net is the current system of development assistance. However, this system is fatally flawed, not only in the way it is programmed, but in the inadequacy of its extent, and because its allocation is unrelated to levels of poverty. Less than 7 per cent of global aid is spent on human priority concerns of basic education, primary health care, family planning, safe drinking water and nutritional programs. Only a quarter of overseas aid flow is earmarked for the ten countries containing three-fourths of the world's absolute poor. In fact, India, Pakistan and Bangladesh contain nearly one-half of the world's poor but get only one-tenth of total aid.

Twice as much development assistance per capita is given to high military spenders among the developing world as to more moderate military spenders. The international financial institutions, like the World Bank and the IMF, are now taking more money out of the developing world than they are putting in, adding to the reverse transfer of around $50 billion per year to the commercial banks.

If overseas aid is to be able to serve as a social safety net for the world's poor, it will have to be based on principles requiring that aid should be directed to priority concerns for human survival and human development.

These four social contracts or partnerships are essential to an effective sustainable response to this epidemic. They will be difficult to forge and will not come about without the commitment and courage of our leaders and friends. There is an ever increasing urgency to embark upon the endeavor to build them.

Conclusion: The Way

At the heart of this epidemic, either there can be violence and fragmentation or there can be stillness. In the hearts of those yet personally untouched by it, it is the

same. It is the same in the hearts of those affected. For all of us, knowing how to
live with HIV can bring a certain stillness to the center of our lives. It can still the
violence and the fragmentation, the fear and the denial. It is this stillness which
creates the possibility of living.

We need to reach out to each other, as one human being to another. There can
be no Them and Us if this epidemic is to be overcome. We are all seeking to pass
from untruth to truth, from darkness to light, from vulnerability to ease. There is a
special truth and light, a special love and laughter, which can be given to us by
those who are courageous enough to tell their stories. We must learn to share in
their sadness and hope, their tears and laughter. We must partake of their dignity
and courage.

We are engaged upon a voyage of understanding. This voyage will require from
each of us truth, compassion, faith, wisdom, respect for others and courage. It will
be a voyage of understanding what is, of understanding reality, not of asserting what
we would like to be the case, what we would prefer to believe.

It will be a voyage of sharing, the sharing of a sense of mystery, of a burden of
sadness, of the pain of care, of the laughter of life. It will be a voyage to change for
each of us, for none of us are untouched by this epidemic. It will be a voyage of the
heart and the mind to communities of concern and commitment. It will be a voyage
through pain, through the dark side of the epidemic, with hope.

11

Placing Women at the Center of Analysis

Elizabeth Reid

There is a growing consensus in the development assistance world that human development should provide the framework for development assistance in the 1990s. Yet, while this is widely welcomed by women, there are few, if any, grounds for assuming that this ideology will benefit women any more than any of the previous development assistance ideologies, be they economic growth, growth with equity, basic needs or whatsoever.

The literature on women and development extends back almost as far as the literature on development itself. The mandates and directives have long been in place. Yet, the success stories are anecdotal rather than systemic and this is causing a growing questioning of past approaches.

There are those amongst us, serious but with a sense of humor, who, in response to this chronic failure, are now proposing two new but linked approaches: the radical procedural approach and the radical analytical approach. The first approach consists in developing a set of procedures that might better bring about the achievement of our women in development objectives. For example, all missions that are responsible for programme or project formulation, implementation teams and evaluation missions must be predominantly or exclusively composed of women. All those consulted during such missions must be predominantly or exclusively women, and so on. Such procedural directives, if issued by United Nations Development Programme (UNDP) or Canadian International Development Agency (CIDA), for example, would undoubtedly be greeted by great discomfiture if not outrage. But it is interesting to note that the obverse, which is the present situation, is not.

The radical analytical approach places women at the center of the analysis; that is, in any development-related activity whatsoever, the analysis should begin at where women are, whatever they are doing, and should aim to get them (women) where they want to be and bring about the changes they want. The rest of the world (men, children, social institutions, financial institutions, economies, etc.) are to be drawn into the analysis primarily on the basis of how they relate to women or how they can contribute to achieving women's goals. Again, radical only in that the obverse is the accepted *modus operandi.*

Today is not the occasion to elaborate on these approaches, but it is the occasion to understand the cost if we do not place women at the center of the HIV analysis. The failure to do so has already brought an immense cost in women's lives, a cost which is forcing an understanding that, for the 1990s and beyond, human development will be conditional upon human survival; that is, human survival, not human development, may well become the primary focus of our development assistance.

Let me elaborate on this, taking the example of HIV. The main focus of HIV programmes to date has been the prevention of the further transmission of the virus. I will focus on sexual transmission since, for women, this is the overwhelming way in which women become infected.

The three main prevention strategies for sexual transmission that are being advocated, particularly in developing countries, are: one, the reduction of the number of sexual partners; two, condom usage; and three, faithfulness in relationships and celibacy and abstinence outside of them. To these, a fourth has recently been added, namely, the treatment of STDs. I do not wish to discuss, today, the merits of these strategies, per se, but rather to look at their adequacy as prevention strategies for women and those who people women's world.

Let's take the first, reduction of sexual partners. Preliminary data from African studies indicate that 60 to 80% of all infected women have one and only one sexual partner. Therefore, this strategy has no relevance to the lives of most of them. It is not relevant to the lives of those women who, because of economic circumstances, are forced to sell or exchange sexual intercourse. Thus, for the majority of women this strategy is inapplicable, irrelevant strategy.

Second, is condom usage. Men use condoms. Results from programmes with sex workers have clearly shown that some women can successfully negotiate condom use. However, this remains a rare skill among women. Most men do not use condoms, and most women do not have the ability or the leverage to protect themselves in this way. This is a strategy for men.

Third, are faithfulness, abstinence and celibacy. At the current stage of the epidemic, it can be estimated that every day, each day now, 1,500 faithful women, are infected. That is, every day, just now, there are 1,500 women who have no sexual partners other than their husbands who are becoming infected. This number will increase as the number of infected men increases. There are some indications that the incidence of rape, particularly of young girls, has increased and there is no reason to believe, in fact, on the contrary, that this is not also true of incest. For most women, abstinence and the faithfulness of both partners in a relationship is not within their power to bring about. For a growing number of girls and women, sexual assault is a reality. So this strategy is inapplicable.

These are grim facts. But they are the realities that lie hidden behind the epidemiological data. The strategies that are being advocated are strategies that men, not women, have under their control. This is the reason why one in every 40 adult women in Africa is infected. It is the reason why there are as many or more infected women in Africa than men. It is also the reason why, in the Latin American and Caribbean regions, the male/female infection ratio has dropped so precipitously over the last couple of years.

Is there no hope for women? In the longer term, the power imbalances in relationships and society which create women's subordination must be changed. But what, in the short term, can women do to save their lives and those of their children?

If one lays aside for the moment the current strategies and begins the analysis with the reality of women's lives, then the first question is: Is there any protective measure that a woman has under her own control which will offer her protection from infection?

Protective measures can be divided into two types: those which prevent contact with an infected person and transmission of the virus and those that decrease the efficacy of transmission when unprotected sexual contact occurs. The first, for example, includes condom usage, faithfulness and abstinence. These measures are much more efficacious than the second type. However, the second type may overall be just as effective, or more effective, if more people can act upon them.

There are, in fact, in each of these two categories, some measures that an individual woman can use. It is important that we start naming them. One of the most efficient known means of reducing the efficacy of transmission of the virus, that is, when you have unprotected sexual intercourse with an infected person, is unbroken genital skin. This is the advice we give to health workers: The most effective barrier is unbroken skin. If you are covered in blood, wash it off. In the genital area, unbroken skin is also protective.

Transmission of the virus can be facilitated by the presence of genital lesions, inflammation, secretions and scarification. The causes of these conditions in women include genital urinary tract infections, sexually transmitted diseases (STDs), sexual practices and traditional infibulation practices. All genital conditions which may facilitate transmission should now become a focus of attention. Not all of them do women have the power to change. A number are treatable. Others, in particular, sexual and infibulation practices, will require longer term solutions. However, there are many conditions that can be improved, through improved hygiene or through treatment.

Women may be culturally or socially constrained from using STD-dedicated services, or even from seeking treatment for a genital condition. This is often not culturally or socially sanctioned. If we want to enable women to avail themselves of this means of protection, it becomes important to know whether the diagnosis and treatment of these conditions can be combined, for example, with other consultations requiring an internal examination. That is, if women cannot go to be treated for these conditions, can we locate services where they are already being externally examined.

This analysis will lead to a broader emphasis on, then an exclusive focus on improving STD services. STD services are mainly used by people, men and women, with multiple sexual partners. Most women do not use these services and most women suffer from genital conditions other than, but also including, STDs. Thus, a woman-centered analysis in this area would focus on the diagnosis and treatment of those genital conditions in both men and women which place them at increased risk of infection and would focus on the delivery of services at points where these people go.

Another strategy for reducing the efficacy of transmission may be to ensure that the changes in a person's infectivity over the course of infection are widely known. A person's infectiousness, the ability to infect someone else, increases as he or she progresses from asymptomatic infection to symptomatic infection. Whereas an individual woman may not be able to refuse sexual intercourse in general, she may be able to find a way if her partner were ill. In other words, she may be able to do this in a short period of time although not over a long period of time. This knowledge about infectivity is an important element in the counseling of discordant couples in our societies. In societies where the virus is diffused throughout the population, this information should be widely known so that those who can, can use it as a protective measure.

Apart from the above, there are at least two strategies for preventing contact with an infected person, the first type of measure, which are under a woman's control. Little attention has been given to barrier methods which, unlike the condom, are under a woman's control. The literature on the sexual transmission of diseases other than HIV to women indicate that diaphragms protect women from, for example, gonorrhea, to the same extent that condom usage does. There is no reason to assume that condoms protect women more than diaphragms do, with or without a spermicide, in the case of HIV. Yet, no attention has been given to determining the adequacy of diaphragms as a protective measure.

The second strategy under women's control for preventing contact with an infected man is, in the absence of any known alternatives, becoming more widespread in high incidence areas. This is desertion. That is, just moving away, walking away from home and relationship. It is an option often with tragic consequences for the woman who may well find herself unable to support herself and, when she is able to take them, her children. In such cases, prostitution, and so infection, may be her only coping strategy.

There is a pressing need to further explore and identify the strategies which a woman may have under her control. However, at the same time it must be understood that the most efficient and effective prevention strategies are those that men have under their control. Thus, every effort must continue to be made to change men's behavior.

In this area, also, there has been a great neglect of a woman-centered analysis. There are at least two very powerful instruments that have not yet been fully identified in the efforts to change men's behavior. The first is women's collective action. The second is the law.

While women individually may feel and be powerless to change men's behavior, women collectively can effect extraordinary changes. The literature on the global movement of women over the last couple of decades abounds with examples. The women of Maharastra who decided to no longer tolerate drunkenness in men, in their husbands, formed themselves into vigilante groups. As a group, not individually, they went out looking for the stills and for drunken men. They changed drinking men's drinking patterns. The Chipko women tied themselves to trees to prevent environmental degradation in Nepal. Mexican women in the mid- to late seventies formed an alliance across all types of women and women's groups to bring down the incidence of rape and sexual assault of women. Kenyan women, also tired of drunkenness in their husbands, came together to devise strategies for stopping that behavior. And the models go on and on.

There is a need to look for models of women's collective action which have changed men's HIV-related behavior. The collective voices and actions of women to be called upon can range from the national machineries for women and national women's organizations, all the way to groupings of women at the village level. We learnt in Kenya that if you wish to increase women's income, you cannot give a goat to a woman. Traditionally, goats are owned by men. If you give a goat to a woman, the man will slaughter it when he chooses and take the money. What the women did, then, was to come collectively together. If women collectively owned a goat, no individual husband could make such a decision. We need analogues to face this epidemic.

The second instrument is the law. There is now an extremely effective and very active Women and Law project in southern Africa. At the initiation of this project and for quite different reasons, it was decided that one important area of study would be the newly introduced laws relating to child support. These laws required men to pay for the upkeep of any children that they fathered. What the Women and Law project has found is that there have been striking changes in male sexual behavior. Men are now fathering fewer children. Now that they are required to provide for and support those that they father, they father fewer.

This provides an important model. We have tried for a long time through direct legal interventions in the area of rape and incest to change men's behavior but with varied success. Here is an example of the use of the law to bring about behavior change which has been extremely effective.

While the primary analysis so far has focused on prevention, a similar analysis is needed to determine the potential impact of this epidemic on individual families, communities and economies and, hence, to plan effective and timely responses. Even in, so to speak, the male-centered analysis, we are not very far along the road to understanding, describing and finding effective strategies. But the point I am making is that what we need to do is to start elsewhere, in this area too, to start in women's spaces.

Let me give you some glimpses of what a woman-centered analysis would reveal. First, most women do not know that they are infected. Most women do not want to know. Infected or otherwise, they must still continue with their daily lives. There is no one to take their place.

For many women who know that they are infected, there is no privacy, no confidentiality. Disclosure is not in their hands. Most women find out that they are infected during pregnancy or when a young child falls ill and is diagnosed. The diagnosis of the child makes public the women's infection status.

For women who know that they are infected, what dominates virtually every minute of the day are two primary emotions: anger and guilt. Anger towards the person, usually their husband and the person with whom they share their daily lives, who infected them. And guilt because they have so often infected one or more of their children.

The reality of the lives of these women is that, although, as stated above, probably up to 60 or 80% of infected women were not infected through their own behavior, they are blamed as the source of the transmission. The stigma and the discrimination associated with this disease rests too often with women.

Next, the supportive services required by seropositive women will be more than drugs and medical care. They will range from household care for ill women, child care for their children, emotional support to deal with anger and guilt, social support to deal with stigma, legal support to lessen discrimination, and financial support, as so often they will not have an income coming into the house. The dominant concern for many infected women is the present and future support for and care of their children, particularly since the fathers of those children will often be sick or dead.

The displacement of women's work from parenting, from productive activities and from community work to care for the sick will have immense consequences within those families and communities. This displacement, coupled with the high mortality rates in women, could well lead to the disintegration of family structures. This can be seen already in parts of Africa. It will lead to changing patterns of agricultural production and the possibility of decreased food production, and to a decrease in informal sector trading where women trade mainly food. It will lead to shortages of personnel in those formal sectors where women predominate, which still include health and education.

If one includes in one's analysis of the HIV epidemic an analysis centered on women, whether it be with respect to prevention or with respect to developing strategies for minimizing the impact of this epidemic, it is my contention that different strategies and priorities will be identified which may end up being more effective than the present strategies. This is not an academic or a feminist exercise. For women, it is a matter of life and death.

Putting women at the center of the analysis leads to quite different approaches and strategies. For women today, the lack of this analysis for the HIV epidemic has already cost perhaps millions of lives, theirs and their children. The price is too high to continue with the blindness of the past. We must change.

12

AIDS from Africa:
A Case of Racism Vs. Science?

Rosalind J. Harrison-Chirimuuta
Richard C. Chirimuuta

Introduction

Western scientists have promoted the hypothesis that the AIDS epidemic began in Africa, arguing that either AIDS had existed for many years in an African "lost tribe" or that a retro virus crossed the species barrier from monkey to man. The scientific evidence in support of this hypothesis has included AIDS-like cases from Africa that predated the epidemic in the West, seroepidermiological evidence for early African infection, and the isolation from African monkeys of retro viruses considered similar to the human immunodeficiency virus. Yet when the scientific literature supporting an African origin is examined it is found to be contradictory, insubstantial or unsound, whilst the possibility that AIDS was introduced to Africa from the West has not been seriously investigated. The belief that the AIDS epidemic originated in Africa has also distorted Western perceptions of the scale and mode of spread of the epidemic in Africa, and it would seem that much of the research into AIDS has been influenced by racism and not science.

The Acquired Immune Deficiency Syndrome (AIDS) was first recognized as a clinical entity in 1981 in the United States (Gottlieb, Shanker and Fan et al. 1981), and although the majority of cases even today have been reported from the United States (WHO 1990b), the Western scientific community has convinced the world that it is primarily an African disease and an African problem. To explain how a disease originating in one continent was yet disseminated to the rest of the world from another, the scientists have argued that there was a remote central African "lost tribe" in whom the virus had been present for centuries (De Cock 1984), or alternatively who acquired the infection from monkeys 30 or so years ago (Hirsch,

165

Olmstead and Murphey-Corb et al. 1989). Haitians (but no one else) working in central Africa then became infected (presumably heterosexually) and, on returning home, spread the disease to homosexual American tourists (Gallo 1987; Farthing, Brown and Staughton 1988). By this circuitous route the virus reached the United States and from there spread to the rest of the world.

Because we suspected a racist motivation for the "science" that was arguing for AIDS from Africa we decided to review the scientific literature, eventually publishing our work in a book (Chirimuuta and Chirimuuta 1989). When questioning the African hypothesis we anticipated a difficult task, as the research was conducted by reputable scientists and was subjected to peer review prior to publication. As our study progressed it became increasingly clear to us that the racist preconceptions of the researchers led them to conclusions that had no scientific foundation.

The Ideology of Racism

It is perhaps unwise to assume a consensus view of racism where none may exist, and for our purposes we would consider racism to be the ideology promoted initially by the Caribbean sugar-planters and slave-merchants to justify, sustain and defend their activities so important to the enrichment of Europe during the 17th and 18th centuries. The ideology was adapted and developed during the period of European colonization during the 19th century and in the 20th century, reaching its apogee in the death camps of Nazi Germany. Unlike the variety of superstitious beliefs Europeans held of other peoples in previous centuries racism was relatively systematic and internally consistent, and with time acquired a pseudo-scientific veneer that glossed over its irrationalities and enabled it to claim intellectual respectability (Fryer 1984). Although the edifice of racism has begun to crack in the latter part of this century, racism remains integral to the European world view.

Many leading doctors and scientists of their day made their contributions to the pseudo-science of racism (Fryer 1984; Ferguson 1984). When humans were placed at the top of the evolutionary tree, Africans were allocated a separate species between other humans and apes and there were numerous suggestions that Africans had sexual intercourse with apes, or were the result of such unions. As Africans were deemed more akin to animals than humans, they were by definition incapable of civilized behavior. They were believed to be sexually unrestrained and to have larger sexual organs than other races, and were therefore more prone to sexually transmitted diseases. They were deceitful, treacherous, lazy, faithless, cruel and bad-tempered. African skulls were studied and were considered to be smaller than those of Europeans, establishing beyond doubt that Africans had the lesser intelligence. In one form or another, explicitly or implicitly, many of these notions have appeared in the scientific literature about AIDS and Africa.

Racism and "AIDS from Africa"

The first black people diagnosed as suffering from AIDS in any number were Haitians living in the United States (*MMWR* 1982; Viera, Frank, Spira et al. 1983), and without serious consideration of the possibility that they might have caught the infection from Americans in Haiti or the United States, Haiti was immediately accused of being the source of the epidemic (Viera et al. 1983). Soon Haitians with AIDS were being reported from all over the Western world (Andreani, Le Charpentier, Brouet et al. 1983; Dournin, Penalba, Wolfe et al. 1983; Autran, Gorin, Leibowitch et al. 1983; The Advisory Group on AIDS 1986), and the Centers for Disease Control (CDC) in Atlanta, Georgia, included Haitians as a group at risk of AIDS along with homosexuals, intravenous drug users and hemophiliacs. It was only in 1985 that CDC, faced with overwhelming evidence that Haitians per se were no more at risk from AIDS than anyone else (Pichenik, Spira, Elie et al. 1985), removed them from the high risk classification but not before Haitians *en masse* were dismissed from their jobs, evicted from their homes, and even housed in separate prisons. Abandoning Haiti, the researchers then turned their attention to Africa.

One of the reasons given by scientists for this turn to Africa was the high incidence of Kaposi's sarcoma (KS) in Africa, although it was clear from the beginning that the benign course of African KS was very different from the aggressive, disseminated form of KS in AIDS patients (Bayley1983). A number of AIDS-like cases were reported retrospectively, the most cited being Dr Rask, a Danish surgeon who worked in Zaire and died in 1977 (Bygbjerg 1983). This patient was given prominence in the best selling-book by Randy Shilts "And The Band Played On," where, under "Dramatis Personae" she is listed as "Danish surgeon in Zaire, first Westerner to have died of AIDS," and is described in the following manner:

> The battle between humans and disease was nowhere more bitterly fought than here in the fetid equatorial climate, where heat and humidity fuel the generation of new life forms . . . Here, on the frontiers of the world's harshest realities, Grethe Rask tended the sick (Shilts 1987).

Jonathan Mann, former director of the AIDS program for the World Health Organization (WHO) and medical text books cite the case as evidence that AIDS originated in central Africa (Mann 1987; Koch-Weiser and Vanderschmidt 1989). It was claimed that Dr. Rask acquired the infection from her patients, at least one of whom had KS, but there was no firm evidence that she died of AIDS, and other diagnostic possibilities were not considered. In 1988, five years after the case was published, we learned that her serum had been tested and found human immunodeficiency virus (HIV) enzyme liked immunosorbent assay (ELISA) negative (Bygbjerg 1988), but the author of the original paper has not published this information in the scientific literature.

Although such AIDS-like cases are presented as evidence that the human immunodeficiency virus existed in Africa prior to the American epidemic, only African cases are considered and the many instances of AIDS-like cases documented in Europe and America (Katner and Pankey 1987) are conveniently ignored. Indeed, on the opposite page to the report of the Danish surgeon in the same issue of the Lancet was an account of an AIDS-like illness in young German homosexual (Sterry, Marmor, Konrads et al. 1983), but whilst non-AIDS in a Danish surgeon heads the citation index proving an African origin, the German case has rarely, if ever, been cited.

The next source of support for the African hypothesis came from the seroepidemiological studies undertaken in Africa or on African serum stored in the West. This research, more than any other, has been at the foundation of all the fantastic stories of millions dying in Africa. Using an enzyme linked immunosorbent assay seropositive figures of 25% of patients attending a clinic in rural Zaire in 1984 (Biggar, Melbye, Kestens et al. 1985), 50% of the Turkanas in Kenya from 1980-1984 (Biggar, Johnson, Oster et al. 1985), and 66% of children in Uganda in 1972 (Saxinger, Levine, Dean et al. 1985) were reported. As AIDS was rare or unknown in the areas where the serum was collected, one would expect the authors to have had serious doubts about the reliability of the tests but, sadly, scientific skepticism has never been a feature of AIDS research in Africa.

One of the most cited studies was undertaken on serum collected in Zaire in 1959 (Nahmias, Weiss, Yao et al. 1986). Using a number of tests in addition to ELISA, only one of 1213 plasmas was positive, but the identity of the donor, described as "rural Bantu", was no longer known. As with the sporadic AIDS-like cases, only seroepidemiology in Africa is considered relevant to the question of the origin of HIV. A study using the same tests was undertaken on stored serum from "aboriginal" Amazonian Indians in Venezuela in 1968/69 and 9 of 224 samples were positive on all the tests (Rodriquez, Sinangil, Volsky et al. 1985). The results were challenged by other researchers as probable false positivity (Biggar 1986a), but the single positive sample from Zaire continues to be cited as evidence that the world AIDS epidemic began in Zaire 35 years ago.

In an interview shown on British television, Professor Hunsmann, head of virology and immunology section and professor of medicine at the German Center of Primate Research at Gottingen, discussed the problems of seroepidemiology:

> We had conducted quite extensive experiments in respect to the epidemiology... of the first human retro virus . . . HTLV [Human T-Lymphotropic Virus]-1 . . . For this reason we had several thousand serum samples frozen and saved in our refrigerated stock. When the news came that there was another, and new human retro virus discovered, the AIDS virus . . . we could immediately search among our stock and probe for an earlier presence of this virus in Africa . . . These tests quickly and clearly gave results, namely, that the first "positive" probes which we could find among our more than 7,000 serum samples are dated only after the beginning of the eighties, from the years 1982-83; and that among samples from before that date—and we had quite a lot of that earlier in our stock—not a single one proved positive. We have

concluded from all this that most other researchers had probably fallen victim to the technical difficulties connected with the conservation and analysis of older serum samples. And the American authors who originally had produced those high percentage data had to correct them—but certainly, once some wrong information like that has been put into circulation, it continues to go on. This has lead to quite a lot of friction between some African states and the United States (Hunsmann 1990).

Later in the same interview when asked why AIDS is not considered to have originated in the United States, Professor Hunsmann made the following comment:

Testing of the kind being done in Africa and to that volume has never been done by anyone in America. Nobody has looked at the stocked blood serum in the USA and there certainly is much more there than in Africa. Nor has anyone asked what happened to the general population. Only one single group, the homosexual community in San Francisco has been analysed and the results showed a high percentage of HIV positivity already by the mid 1970's. But no other samples have been tested to the extent done in Africa. I think this should be clearly said (Hunsmann 1990).

Why, then, if this research is valid (and there have been serious criticisms) have other AIDS researchers persisted in arguing that the African AIDS epidemic preceded the epidemic elsewhere in the world? And if the tests are unreliable, why are the predictions that millions of Africans will soon die from AIDS still presented without comment? How, indeed, is it possible that a virus could spread so much more rapidly by heterosexual contact in Africa than anywhere else in the world? It is here as in so many other aspects of AIDS research, that racist beliefs about the sexual propensities and promiscuity of Africans conflict with scientific evidence, and in such a confrontation belief is almost invariably the victor.

Researchers had originally proposed that AIDS was an "old disease of Africa" that had reached the West via recent intercontinental travel (De Cock 1984) a rather curious notion given the enforced intercontinental travel of up to 100 million Africans in previous centuries (Davidson 1978). As this hypothesis became increasingly untenable attention was diverted to the possibility of a monkey origin of the virus. Such ideas cohabit easily with racist notions that Africans are evolutionarily closer to sub-human primates. Dr Robert Gallo and his co-workers were among the pioneers of this line of research, both for HTLV-I and HTLV-III (later renamed HIV) (Gallo 1987; Gallo, Sliski and Wong-Staal 1983; Gallo 1986). Two of Gallo's colleagues, Kanki and Essex, reported the isolation of a virus similar to HTLV-III in macaque monkeys who were suffering from an AIDS-like illness, and labeled it simian T-Lymphotropic virus type III (STLV-III) of macaques (Daniel, Letvin, Kanki et al. 1985). For those who were arguing an African origin of the AIDS virus, an Asian monkey like the macaque was not a suitable source but less than 6 months later the same researchers reported finding the virus in "wild-caught" African green monkeys from Kenya and Ethiopia (Kanki, Alroy and Essex 1985). This research was motivated only by a desire to believe an African origin of the disease, and was greeted with enthusiasm by the western scientific community. Discussion quickly moved on to the question of how the virus crossed the species barrier, and two AIDS "experts" from St Mary's Hospital in London even offered this explanation:

> Monkeys are often hunted for food in Africa. It may be that a hunting accident of some sort, or an accident in preparation for cooking, brought people in contact with infected blood. Once caught, monkeys are often kept in huts for some time before they are eaten. Dead monkeys are sometimes used as toys for African children (Green and Miller 1986).

Are we seriously to believe that African parents are so desperate for toys for their children that they give them putrefying carcasses of dead animals? More fantastic suggestions were published in *The Lancet:*

> Sir:- The isolation from monkeys of retro viruses closely related to HIV strongly suggests a simian origin for this virus . . . Several unlikely hypotheses have been put forward . . . In his book on the sexual life of people of the Great Lakes area of Africa Kashamura writes: "pour stimuler intense, on leur inocule dans les cuisses, la region du pubis et le dos du sang preleve sur un singe, pour un homme, sur une guenon, pour le femme" (to stimulate a man or a woman and induce them to intense sexual activity, monkey blood [for a man] or she-monkey blood [for a woman] was directly inoculated in the pubic area and also the thighs and back). These magic practices would therefore constitute an efficient experimental transmission model and could be responsible for the emergence of AIDS in man (Noireau 1987).

This came in for particular derision at the conference on AIDS in Africa held at Naples in October 1987:

> When queried regarding the plausibility of a premise put forth in a letter to *The Lancet* suggesting that a bizarre tribal ritual of injecting monkey blood into the pubic region of young African men and women to stimulate intense sexual activity could be responsible for the emergence of AIDS in man, researchers from Zaire, Congo, and Belgium were unanimous in declaring it to be preposterous . . . (*Skin and Allergy News* 1988).

It is hardly surprising that western AIDS researchers and journalists have become persona non grata in many African countries.

Most Africans, in fact, have little contact with monkeys (Biggar 1986b), and amongst those who regularly hunt monkeys, for example the pygmies of the equatorial rain forests, AIDS is notable for its absence (Konotey-Ahulu 1987). On the other hand, in recent years there has been a marked increase in contact between man and monkeys not in Africa but in the West. In the 1920's the transplantation of monkey testes to humans was widely practiced, and many thousands of men in Europe, America and Australia received the benefit of this operation that promised to restore their youth and vigor (Hamilton 1986). Monkeys have also been used widely for scientific research, and with the discovery that their kidneys provide excellent tissue culture material for virus isolation, propagation and vaccine production, hundreds of thousands have been caught and transported from their native haunts (Vella 1977). If there is any truth in the hypothesis that HIV originated in monkeys (and African monkeys are not the only candidates) it would seem more appropriate to investigate modern medical research than speculate about the customs and behavior of Africans.

Although the African green monkey hypothesis was widely accepted, it came under increasing scientific challenge. Attempts to repeat the Essex and Kanki experiments on other wild African green monkeys were unsuccessful (Mulder 1988a), and the genetic sequences of the virus isolated from laboratory macaque monkeys, the virus Essex and Kanki claimed to have isolated from "wild-caught" green monkeys and another supposedly human virus called HTLV-IV, were found to be identical (Kestler, Li, Naidu et al. 1988). Essex and Kanki were then obliged to admit that their green monkey virus was a laboratory contaminant (Essex and Kanki 1988). A retro virus was eventually isolated from African green monkeys, but it bore little resemblance either to the macaque virus or the human AIDS viruses, and could not have originated from African green monkeys in recent times (Mulder 1988b; Fukasawa, Miura, Hasegawa et al. 1988). It is difficult to understand why this virus has been called simian immunodeficiency virus of African green monkeys (SIVagm) as it does not cause immune deficiency. In all this confusion of viruses one question surely needs to be asked: What is the origin of the virus that caused AIDS-like illnesses in laboratory macaque monkeys? This virus does not occur in wild macaque monkeys, but does have some similarity with the human AIDS viruses. Had these monkeys been subjected to experiments with retro viruses, and did the appearance of AIDS-like illnesses in the monkeys predate the human AIDS epidemic?

It is instructive for anyone who still has illusions about the objectivity of science or the integrity of some AIDS researchers to read the October 1988 edition of *Scientific American*. The issue was devoted to AIDS, and the section titled "The Origins of the AIDS Virus" was written by Essex and Kanki and was illustrated by a full page color photograph of an African green monkey. Eight months after admitting that the African green monkey virus was a laboratory contaminant, Essex and Kanki had the audacity to state:

> Why SIV is endemic in these African monkeys but seems to do them no harm, and is also found in the captive Asian macaques, where it causes disease, was (and still is) enigma...(Essex and Kanki 1988b).

Does this re-presentation of discredited data signal the abandonment of any pretence of scientific integrity in order to promote conscious and deliberate propaganda?

Other attempts to implicate Africa in the AIDS epidemic also came to grief. Dr. Anthony Pinching and his team from St Mary's Hospital, London, claimed that a particular genetic variant, the Gcf allele, predisposed the person to infection with HIV, and that this variant was common in central Africa (Eales, Parkin, Pinching et al. 1987). The Gcf allele had, in fact, been found to be common in the Bi Aka pygmies of the Central African Republic and the Peuhl Fula of Sengal, ethnically distinct groups in whom AIDS was either rare or absent (Konotey-Ahulu 1987), but it would seem to European minds all Africans are the same and somehow genetically distinct from other races. This research was reported in the media as a major breakthrough in the search for a cure for AIDS (Konotey-Ahulu 1987), but a year later, after a number of other laboratories failed to confirm the findings, Dr. Pinching admitted that their original data was erroneous (Eales, Nye, and Pinching 1988). At least Dr. Pinching, unlike Dr. Bygbjerg and so many other AIDS researchers, had the courtesy to admit his error publicly and apologies to his fellow scientists for the extra work he had caused, although his apologies were not extended to the many Africans whom he had offended.

Although many AIDS researchers now appreciate that they have offended and angered many black people, they remain ignorant of their unconscious racism and continue to give offence. The September 1988 edition of *Medicine International* was devoted to the subject of AIDS, and as usual there was an article on AIDS in Africa, but no similar discussion about AIDS in any other continent. The authors commented on the problems created by earlier AIDS research in Africa:

> Initial claims that the disease had been present in Africa for long enough for widespread immunity to have developed in exposed populations were false; epidemics of AIDS were as new in Africa as elsewhere. Considerable damage has been done to international research collaboration as a result of these claims (Nunn and McAdam 1988).

But later in the same article:

> The scale of African AIDS epidemic has led to speculation that heterosexual transmission is more efficient in Africa than elsewhere . . . Social and cultural factors, such as the African tradition of male sexual freedom, may also play a part. The circulation of myths such as the only cure for AIDS being to have sex with a virgin is likely to have a greater effect on transmission in Africa than in developed countries (Nunn and McAdam 1988).

What do the authors of this paper know about African traditions of male sexual freedom, and does no such "tradition" exist in the West? And on what evidence are we to believe that a significant number of African men are having sex with virgins to cure themselves of AIDS? But then if you already believe that Africans are more primitive and superstitious no evidence is required.

Other AIDS researchers have recognized that their past activities have caused problems. *The British Medical Bulletin* of January 1988, titled "AIDS and HIV infection: the wider perspective," was edited by three notable exponents of the

African connection, Anthony Pinching, Robin Weiss and David Miller. They provide a classic example of muddled racist thinking:

> In the case of some early studies in Africa, techniques were used that had not been sufficiently well validated for African sera . . . The observations derived from these studies have led to some confusion and have also tended to damage the credibility of foreign scientists working in Africa—especially among local leaders (Piot and Carael 1988b).

Who was confused by this bad science? Certainly not Africans, whether ordinary citizens or "local leaders". The racist themes were all too familiar, the response was anger and not confusion, and the discrediting of the science came as no surprise, as it was never believed in the first place. The AIDS experts continue:

> Additional problems have been created when investigators have spent a short time collecting sera and basic data in a developing country, often with little guidance from local investigators, and then published the data without reference to the original context. This has tended to produce scientific data that have not been adequately placed in an anthropological perspective (Piot and Carael 1988).

In other words data collection was biased or inadequate, and this led to a misinterpretation of results. The racism responsible for this is charmingly described as an inadequate "anthropological perspective!" But worse is to come:

> Even worse, it has led to denial and resentment, jeopardizing essential and potentially fruitful collaboration between investigators in the developed and developing world in the study of mutual concern. This has been particularly damaging when the pursuit has apparently been the origin of AIDS and HIV, an essentially academic question, however interesting. Such investigations have often been taken to imply blame on the region that appears to be the source. Although they were certainly never intended to impugn any community in this way, it was not difficult to see how such perceptions arose (Piot and Carael 1988).

Recognition that the faulty techniques described at the beginning of the paragraph provided the "evidence" for an African origin for HIV is beyond the wit of these clever scientists, who then accuse Africans of "denial and resentment" when they refuse to accept their findings! Let us gratefully accept their condolences for the injuries they have inflicted, and put aside our resentments, so that we can leave ourselves open to more of the same, to be found later in the Bulletin:

> HIV infection appears to have spread over much of the world during the decade 1976-1986, mirroring on a large scale the spread of its most obvious predecessor, syphilis, in Europe in the 1490's. As with early syphilis, the international spread of AIDS has led to a process of attribution and denial about the origin of the disease. However, it seems most likely that HIV spread to the United States from Africa,

perhaps via Haiti, in the mid 1970's and from the United States to many western countries in the late 1970's and early 1980's (Moss 1988).

Others are not so confident, at least when they address Africans at AIDS and Africa conferences:

> Luc Montaigner, the first scientist to isolate the virus that causes AIDS, agrees that if an isolated population in Africa existed as a reservoir for the virus, researchers would have found it by now. The data suggesting that the virus comes from Africa are weak, Montaigner said "Maybe we should look to another part of the world" (*New Scientist* 1987).

Jonathan Mann, then the director of WHO's AIDS program, also felt obliged to distance himself from an African origin:

> The World Health Organization's position is that there is not yet enough information about the origin of the virus. There are absolutely no data to support any hypothesis... "The more information that emerges, the less we know about where this virus came from, how long it has been in the world, and how it grew to become the problem that it is today, " he said. The syndrome has too often unveiled thinly disguised prejudices about race, religion, sex, social class, and nationality, and the Africans properly resent that Africa has been singled out, Dr. Mann said. If San Francisco was accused of being the original source of HIV with no more proof than there is that Africa is the source, special interest groups would be up in arms, he said . . . Dr. Mann said nothing will keep people from coming up with "cheap hypotheses" about the origin of AIDS. "They die a natural death when no subsequent evidence develops to take them seriously. But journals should have a special page for them labeled 'fuzzy ideas', he said. "The real danger is that future authors might use such discredited, but published, hypotheses as scientific references for future articles", he said (*Skin and Allergy News* 1988).

This would seem a classic case of white man speaking with forked tongue, as there is qualitative difference between racism and mere "fuzzy ideas", and whilst the publication of "fuzzy ideas" may be no more than a reflection of the quality of the journal, racism should find no place in its pages. The director of the WHO's AIDS program and his associates were in a position to request that the medical and scientific journals adopt and implement anti-racist policies. Instead they were content to show their bleeding hearts only at conferences attended by Africans.

Although racism can be found in abundance in the medical literature about AIDS and Africa, two psychologists, J. Phillipe Rushton and Anthony F. Bogaert, have drawn together these ideas and have attempted to give them a pseudo-scientific coherence. According to the British newspaper *The Independent on Sunday* Rushton has received funding from a racist American trust and was investigated by the Canadian police under the hate propaganda laws. Rushton and Bogaert's paper, titled "Population differences in susceptibility to AIDS: an evolutionary analysis", was published in a leading British journal, *Social Science and Medicine*. The abstract is as follows:

Previously we have reported population differences in sexual restraint such that, higher socio-economic status > lower socio-economic status, and Mongoloids > Caucasoid's > Negroids. This ordering was predicted from a gene-based evolutionary theory of r/K reproductive strategies in which a trade-off occurs between gamete production and social behaviors such as intelligence, law abindingness, and parental care. Here we consider the implications of these analyses for sexual dysfunction, including susceptibility to AIDS. We conclude that relative to Caucasians, populations of Asian ancestry are inclined to a greater frequency of inhibitory disorders such as low sexual excitement and premature ejaculation and to a lower frequency of sexually transmitted diseases including AIDS, while populations of African ancestry are inclined to a greater frequency of uninhibited disorders such as rape and unintended pregnancy and to more sexually transmitted diseases including AIDS (Rushton and Bogaert 1989).

It is not possible to discuss this article in detail, but the only difference in substance from the pseudo-scientific racism of previous centuries is the different ranking order of the races. Mongoloids are now superior to Caucasoids, although Negroids, of course, remain at the bottom. Meaningless algebraic presentations such as r/K only give a modern veneer to very old ideas. We are told, for example, that the average cranial capacity of Mongoloids is 1448 cm^3 v 1334 cm^3 for Negroids whilst genitalia and secondary sex characteristics of Mongoloids are, of course, small and that of Negroids large, and for such reasons AIDS is rampaging through Africa. It is difficult to believe that such an article would be published anywhere but in a right-wing fringe magazine, but after a decade of AIDS pseudo-science anything seems possible.

The AIDS establishment has typically responded to the charge of racism with the counter accusation that such criticisms deny an African AIDS epidemic, giving African governments an excuse not to take measures to contain the epidemic. In fact we do not deny the existence of an AIDS epidemic in Africa and elsewhere in the world, but believe that the scale of the epidemic is open to question. Whilst doctors from the West claim there are hundreds of thousands of Africans dying from AIDS, and that millions are already infected with HIV, the experience of African doctors and ordinary people is very different. One Zimbabwean woman who in 1988 had not seen or heard or anyone with AIDS said that it was like being asked to believe in the Holy Ghost (*New Scientist* 1988). A Ghanaian physician, Dr Konotey-Ahulu described the AIDS epidemic in the following way:

... The African does not speak of Africa as if it was "a little country somewhere in Timbuktu." Africa is a massive continent with 600 million people in 2,300 tribes distributed in 53 different, sometimes very different, countries. For example, the difference between Ghana and next door Ivory Coast vis a vis the sex trade is the difference between Ghana's ex-colonial master Britain and Cote d'Ivoire's France. Scientific and media descriptions of Africa's "AIDS elephant," with its 53 body parts, have sometimes been like those of the proverbial blind men surveying the elephant. Most researchers concentrate on the tusk and, not surprisingly, come out with "the AIDS problem in Africa is very sharp and pointed; the whole continent is like that." Even when experts from Nigeria, the large body-part of the elephant, confirm with seropositivity studies that there is not yet an AIDS problem in their country, they are shouted down with "Under-reporting Under-reporting! The whole beast has a sharp profile." To these safari experts, Tanzania and Sierra Leone,Uganda and Gabon, Zaire and Ghana, Rwanda and Gambia, are all the same . . . (Konotey-Ahulu 1989).

Dr Konotey- Ahulu toured all the AIDS affected African countries, (except Zaire, where he was refused entry, although US government sponsored AIDS researchers appear to have no such difficulties) and reported his findings in the British Medical Journal and the Lancet:

> In February and March of this year (1987) I made a six-week tour of twenty-six cities and towns in sixteen sub-Saharan countries, including those most afflicted by AIDS, did ward rounds with doctors and nurses, met ministers of health, directors or medical services, and research workers (native and expatriate) . . . If one judges the extent of AIDS in Africa on an arbitrary scale from grade 1 (not much of a problem) to grade V (a catastrophe), in my assessment AIDS is a problem (grade II) in only five, (possibly six, since I was unable to obtain a visa for Zaire) of the countries where AIDS has occurred . . . In no country is the AIDS problem consistently grade III (a great problem), or even grade IV (an extremely great problem), and in none can it be called a catastrophe (grade V). In Kenya, for instance, contrary to widespread reports I would rate AIDS in 1987 as grade I . . . Before the days of AIDS in Ghana there was a death a day...on my ward alone of thirty-four beds . . . They died from one or another of the following: cerebrovascular accident from malignant hypertension, hepatoma, ruptured amoebic abscess, haematemesis, chronic renal failure, sickle-cell crisis, septicaemia, perforated typhoid gut, hepatic coma, haemoptysis from tuberculosis, brain tumor, Hodgkin's disease . . . Today, because of AIDS, it seems that Africans are not allowed to die from these conditions any longer. If tens of thousands are dying from AIDS (and Africans do not cremate their dead) where are the graves? . . . "Why do the world's media appear to have conspired with some scientists to become so gratuitously extravagant with the untruth?"—that was the question uppermost in the minds of intelligent Africans and Europeans I met on my tour (Konotey-Ahulu 1987).

Dr. Konotev-Ahulu was particularly critical of western researchers who, with no experience of tropical medicine, used seroepidemiology as a substitute for, rather than an adjunct to clinical epidemiology, and described the difficulties faced by doctors working in Africa who sought funding from external research agencies to increase their clinical epidemiology research base (Konotey-Ahulu 1987).

Although African governments have repeatedly been accused of under-reporting and the number of AIDS cases notified to the World Health Organization from African countries have never reached the expectations of the Western AIDS establishment, it is important to appreciate how even these relatively modest figures are derived. In the West AIDS is diagnosed and hence reported when a patient develops an opportunistic infection or AIDS dementia (*MMWR* 1987). The diagnosis is confirmed with at least two and often more different types of tests, e.g. ELISA, Western blot, and radioimmuno-precipitation assay. Thus the great majority of patients with symptoms and signs of HIV infection, i.e. those with persistent generalized lymphadenopathy or AIDS related complex (now called symptomatic HIV infection) do not reach the official statistics until they develop opportunistic infections or dementia. There is a degree of under-reporting (up to 20 percent in the United States) but virtually no over-reporting (*MMWR* 1987a). Because of the expense of laboratory tests for HIV infection and opportunistic diseases physicians and health workers in most African states have been encouraged to use the WHO clinical criteria for AIDS, confirmed with ELISA when available (*WHO Weekly Epidemiological Record* 1986). The WHO clinical criteria do not distinguish AIDS and symptomatic HIV infection, and in Africa both are therefore reported as AIDS cases (Berkley, Okware, and Naamara 1989). Nor do they differentiate AIDS from other clinically similar wasting diseases and a number of studies have shown that between 26 and 50 percent of patients who fulfil clinical criteria are seronegative for HIV infection (Jagwe 1986; Colebunders, Francis, Izaley et al. 1987; Nzilambi, De Cock, Forthal et al. 1988).

Diagnostic pitfalls include infections particularly tuberculosis, parasitic infestations, lymphomas and occult carcinomas, and endocrine disorders such as diabetes mellitus, thyrotoxicosis and Addison's disease (Colebunders, Francis, Izaley et al. 1987; Mugerwa 1988). Confirmatory testing with ELISA, if available, also presents difficulties, given the high rate of false positivity with this test, especially in patients already ill from other diseases. In this context it is curious to note that the proportion of African AIDS patients who have died is much lower than that in the West, where it is consistently 50 to 60 percent (*WHO Weekly Epidemiological Record* 1986; Berkley, Okware, and Naamara 1989). It is most unlikely that Africans with AIDS live longer than their Western counterparts, and far more probable that reported African cases include patients at an early stage of the disease and patients with clinically similar but less deadly diseases.

If the criteria used to diagnose AIDS in Africa were used in the West the number of Western AIDS cases would increase manifold, and therefore comparisons between the incidence of AIDS in Africa and the West are meaningless. Such difficulties are usually dismissed on the assumption of enormous under-reporting of AIDS in Africa, but if this were so, what happens to these patients? Do they die, or do they somehow fade away unmourned, unburied and unrecorded. In Africa as in the West AIDS is predominantly afflicting the young, sexually active section of the population and a change in the pattern of disease and death in this group would be reflected in official statistics even if not reported as due to AIDS. This has been demonstrated in Britain where there has been an increase in the death rate amongst young men, and up to 500 may have died of AIDS in the last year without being reported as such (Report from Chief Medical Officer 1990).

Yet Western researchers seem incapable of believing that African countries gather such statistical information although it is often readily available in the libraries of their own institutions. When comparing the incidence of AIDS in different countries, it is important to consider the rate of progression from HIV infection to 'full blown' AIDS. It is probable that this will be more rapid in countries with a high rate of infectious and parasitic disease, and consequently the proportion of AIDS patients to the number with HIV infection will be higher. Even if African states were using the same criteria to diagnose AIDS as in the West, assumptions about the prevalence of HIV infection based on Western experience would be misleading.

Even if one chooses to ignore the information provided by various African Ministries of Health some assessment of the scale of the African epidemic can be made by studying expatriate Africans. Many Africans in Europe and America are temporary residents or travel home frequently, and AIDS in this group should mirror the epidemic in their countries of origin. Whilst there was much excitement about the incidence of AIDS in expatriate Africans in Europe in the early 1980s (Vandepitte, Verwilghen and Zachee 1983; Edwards, Harper and Pain 1984; Brunet, Chaperon, Gluckman et al. 1983) the number of Africans diagnosed in Europe actually declined between 1984 and 1986 (*WHO Weekly Epidemiological Record* 1987), perhaps because reliable tests for AIDS became available, and only in 1987 showed a modest increase. Africans with AIDS in Europe are no longer reported separately by the WHO (*WHO Weekly Epidemiological Record* 1988), perhaps because they have ceased to be a significant proportion of the total European cases. Although there was much talk of the risks of transmission of HIV-2 by West Africans in Britain (Brun-Vezinet, Katlana, and Roulot 1987), more than 6,500 patients with West African connections were tested and all were found negative for this virus (Griffiths and Contreras 1990). It is curious that expatriate Africans in the United States have never featured in discussions about the supposed origin of AIDS, nor have they been reported as suffering from AIDS in any number.

Sound scientific methodology surely dictates that evidence contrary to a proposed hypothesis should be sought as vigorously as evidence for the hypothesis. In the case of AIDS from Africa contrary evidence has not been sought at all, but this singular deficiency in effort is then presented as a lack of result. If scientists did wish to explore the possibility that HIV was introduced to Africa from the United States and Europe we would mention two possible areas for research. The first is the export of infected American blood products. Discussion in the scientific literature about Africa and transmission of HIV by blood products inevitably concentrated on the possible importation of infected plasma to America from Africa (an unsubstantiated hypothesis that died quickly) (Jones 1985) or the spread of HIV in Africa by local blood transfusions (Quinn, Mann, Curran et al. 1986). We could find only one reference to the export of infected America blood to third world countries, in a WHO working paper where it was said that contaminated plasma pools may have been sold at discount prices in developing countries since they could not check the products (Bytchenko 1986). Western countries outside the USA are for the most part self sufficient in whole blood and plasma, and the only significant group infected from America were hemophiliacs who were given imported American clotting factors. Poor countries often cannot afford a blood transfusion service, and wealthy patients with blood loss may be transfused with imported blood whilst the poor at best receive an immediate transfusion from a relative or friend. If imported whole blood or plasma was responsible for introducing AIDS into Africa, this would be consistent with the initial appearance of AIDS in the urban-based elite in countries like Zaire which are particularly dependent on America. It would also account for the development of AIDS in expatriate Europeans, such as the French woman who developed AIDS after a blood transfusion in the Cameroons, as it is unlikely that she was transfused with locally obtained blood (Vittecoq, Roue, Mayaud et al. 1987).

A second, and we suspect far more important route by which AIDS may have been introduced into Africa is sex tourism. AIDS researchers, who seem unable to contemplate that White men can infect African women, have presented AIDS in Africa as a disease transmitted by promiscuous men (and to racist minds all Africans are promiscuous) to prostitutes who then infect foreign clients (Bonneux, Van der Stuyft, Taelman et al. 1988). Prostitution in African countries tends to occur at two levels with younger women seeking valuable foreign exchange who work in the large hotels and night spots which attract foreign tourists and wealthy Africans, and with older women whose clientele is predominantly poor and local. If African realities agreed with research suppositions, older African woman and their local clientele would be bearing the brunt of the epidemic but to the contrary it is the young women frequenting the tourist centers and foreign military and naval establishments who are reported to be developing AIDS and transmitting it to their African sexual partners: husbands, boyfriends and wealthy African clients (*New Scientist* 1988; Neequaye, Neequaye, Mingle et al. 1986).

Conclusion

When discussing the issue of the origin of AIDS we are frequently asked by well meaning people "Does it really matter where AIDS came from, shouldn't we forget about the origin and concentrate on dealing with the epidemic". Certainly we agree that every effort should be made to contain the epidemic, in Africa as elsewhere in the world, but AIDS researchers have opened a Pandora's box of racism and prejudice that cannot be closed by simply dropping the subject of the origin. Incorrect assumptions about the source and nature of the African AIDS epidemic will also inevitably lead to inappropriate programs for containment and control. Africans have complained that scarce resources from the World Health Organization have been diverted from programs to control major epidemic diseases that are killing many more people than AIDS, and insufficient emphasis has been placed on the risks of sex for money whilst the dangers of low levels of promiscuity have been exaggerated to such an extent that people have even committed suicide because they feared they had AIDS.

Although racism in its various manifestations has come under increasing challenge in recent years, it remains a potent influence, and it is naive to believe that medical science is immune to this particular poison. With the emergence of a new and deadly sexually transmitted disease, it was perhaps almost inevitable that Black people would be attributed with its origin and transmission, whatever the evidence. Racism is an irrational system of beliefs without scientific foundation, and much of the confused, contradictory and simply nonsensical conclusions reached by the scientists about AIDS and Africa can be attributed to their attempts to square their research findings with their racist preconceptions. The determined pursuit of the African origin has been of little scientific or practical merit, but instead has escalated racism, created conflict between African and Western countries and diverted resources away from areas where they are much needed, and has wasted time. Let us hope we can learn from our mistakes, otherwise we will be doomed to repeat them.

13

U.S. Aid to AIDS in Africa

Meredeth Turshen

Introduction

The purpose of this communication is to review the assistance provided by the U.S. Government to programs that address the growing problem of acquired immune deficiency syndrome (AIDS) in Africa. The U.S. Agency for International Development (USAID) estimates that 9 million Africans have been infected with the human immunodeficiency virus (HIV) and that two to three million adult AIDS cases are expected in sub-Saharan Africa by the year 2000 (USAID 1993: 8). Approximately $140 million of the more than $400 million obligated by USAID for global HIV/AIDS control from 1987 to 1992 is specifically for Africa (USAID 1993: 14). On the premise that "heterosexual intercourse has been the principal mode of transmission . . . and accounts for over 80 percent of infections," USAID's goal is to decrease the "sexual transmission of HIV by promoting safer sexual behavior using a range of innovative communication strategies," by increasing condom availability and use, and by controlling sexually transmitted diseases (USAID 1993:8, 25). USAID's bilateral program currently provides support for three types of activity: designing and implementing HIV prevention programs, biomedical and behavioral research, and networking for PVOs (private voluntary organizations) (USAID 1993: 15, 19).

U.S. Aid to Africa

It is not possible to document the proportion of the $140 million allocation that was spent in Africa or on supplies that were sent to Africa. Scattered evidence suggests that the proportion is small and that most of the money was spent in the U.S. on suppliers and sub-contractors. Money obligated for condom supplies is spent in the U.S. and the condoms are shipped to Africa, where they are sold or distributed free. Money spent on subcontractors is spent mainly on salaries of personnel based in the U.S. and consultants who travel to Africa. For example, in 1987 USAID granted a five-year $24 million contract to the Washington-based Academy for Educational Development for AIDSCOM, a condom promotion and communication project. AIDSCOM worked in seven African countries—Burundi, Ghana, Malawi, Rwanda, Tanzania, Uganda, and Zambia—which accounted for about one-third of its budget (USAID 1993:15). Another example: from 1988 to 1992, the USAID Bureau for Africa gave $40 million for HIV/AIDS prevention. This project represented one of USAID's first efforts at large-scale funding of PVOs to work in HIV prevention. Five US-based PVOs and one university were funded to conduct nine prevention projects in Africa (USAID 1993:16).

Another US-based nonprofit organization funded by USAID is Family Health International (FHI), which is "dedicated to delivering family planning services worldwide" and headquartered in Triangle Park, North Carolina. FHI's initial five-year project, called AIDSTECH, was concerned with HIV surveillance and screening, blood tests and blood supplies. Three countries—Cameroon, Kenya and Ghana—accounted for half of the $5.2 million obligated to programs in thirty African countries (AIDSTECH/Family Health International 1990). The project has broadened since 1990 to include technical support initiatives, including behavioral change interventions such as peer education in Cameroon, Mali, Niger and Zimbabwe; condom social marketing strategies in Burkina Faso, Cameroon and Zaire; and safer-sex and STD-prevention education initiatives in Burkina Faso (USAID 1993: 16).[1]

In addition to its bilateral aid program, USAID contributed about $100 million to the World Health Organization Global Programme on AIDS from 1986 to 1992 (USAID 1993:14). WHO projects that 8 percent ($150,000) of its small $1.9 million regular budget for AIDS and 19 percent ($33.7 million) of the $180 million special trust fund for the Global Programme on AIDS will be allocated to Africa in 1994-95 (WHO 1992).

These amounts should be read against the reported distribution of AIDS cases worldwide. WHO (1994) recorded a cumulative total of 985,119 cases as of 30 June 1994, 42% (411,907) in the United States and 34% (331,378) in fifty-four African countries. The proportion of US foreign aid earmarked for Africa (35%) is consistent with the extent of the problem. The type of assistance, however, seems inconsistent with the known health problems associated with AIDS and does not take account of worsening health conditions and deteriorating health services in Africa.

Aid is linked to population control and is divorced from health service programs, other than control of sexually transmitted diseases. The type of assistance can be illustrated by HIV prevention activities reported by USAID (1993). In Cameroon and Ghana, the focus is on commercial sex workers and tied to condom promotion and distribution; the same is true of Nigeria, where Family Health International hopes to reach 6,000 commercial sex workers and 100,000 of their partners. Family Health International is targeting high risk behavior groups in Senegal; in Tanzania, the campaign by AMREF targets truck drivers and other transport workers. In Côte d'Ivoire, Population Services International, another U.S PVO, promotes condom use through condom social marketing, short-hand for support to private commercial condom production and distribution.

Examples of assistance to biomedical and behavioral research include a Zambian study of discordant couples (one partner is HIV+ and the other is HIV-), which showed that consistent use of condoms and spermicides substantially reduces the rate of HIV infection in women; a Nigerian project, carried out by the U.S.-based nonprofit International Center for Research on Women, to motivate and foster HIV prevention behaviors among female university students; and a series of studies in Côte d'Ivoire— one to find the HIV seroprevalence rate among secondary school students, a second to assess the impact of AIDS on big business in Abidjan, and a third to study the sexual behavior of youth in the capital.

AIDS education projects may also be divorced from school health and education services. A project in Malawi schools featured government-sponsored focus-group sessions with adolescents; a knowledge, attitude and practice (KAP) survey;[2] and workshops to develop educational materials (USAID 1990: 33-34).

"After three years of research and preparation, more than 250,000 HIV/AIDS prevention textbooks were distributed . . . Despite official support, many school officials, teachers and community leaders remain reluctant to see topics such as sexuality and AIDS prevention introduced in the schools" (USAID 1993: 34).

In other words, despite three years of research and preparation, the textbooks were found objectionable and are not being used. Now the project will sponsor training workshops for teachers and local officials to compel them to cooperate. USAID obligated a total of $615,343 for work in Malawi on this project and on an AIDS reporting system, a government study of the economic impact of AIDS, and a Johns Hopkins University clinical study of the relation between venereal disease and AIDS in women.

Before 1992 Zaire was a major recipient of U.S. aid, but because of the political situation, assistance is now limited to condom supply and promotion. The $2,089,975 obligated for projects in Zaire financed rural field trials of new rapid blood screening tests (which are tests of pooled blood, a clear indication that individuals with AIDS are not a prime concern) carried out by the Program for Appropriate Technology in Health.[3] USAID also funded the promotion of private sector marketing of condoms and a mass media project carried out by Population Services International, which created a social marketing structure to sell condoms donated by USAID at a subsidized price through existing commercial outlets. And USAID funded the creation of an AIDS epidemiology training course set up by the

U.S. National Institutes of Health and Tulane Medical Center at the University of Zaire School of Public Health.

With the $464,362 obligated to Zambia, the Bethesda-based Uniformed Services University of the Health Sciences worked with the University Teaching Hospital in Lusaka to help control sexually transmitted diseases including AIDS in a number of ways: by sponsoring sex education activities in high schools and in the forty-five STD clinics located throughout Zambia; by training nurses, clinical officers, and health administrators in the clinical manifestations of STDs and in the laboratory diagnosis of those infections; by funding a national seminar in Lusaka to instruct 150 health workers who staff STD clinics in techniques for counseling HIV seropositive patients; and by monitoring the health status of more than 10,000 people who are HIV-infected or at risk of becoming infected.

An Analysis of Project Aid

Several points can be made about project aid. First, USAID is channeling funds through U.S.-based private, nonprofit and voluntary organizations, rather than aiding governments or multinational organizations directly.[4] With the disengagement from the UN during the Reagan and Bush administrations, the U.S. began a major shift to the disbursement of funds through private U.S. agencies; the Reagan and Bush administrations preferred private over public initiatives and sought nongovernmental avenues of charitable assistance, believing that "charity begins at home." USAID justifies the shift on the grounds that African governments are corrupt and must be circumvented if aid is to reach its targets. The advantage to this method of disbursement is that it gives the U.S. government more control over funds, as well as the findings of research projects.[5]

Second, many of the PVOs now receiving money for AIDS control were originally founded in the 1970s to halt rapid population growth in the third world. In the past few years, USAID has integrated AIDS control with family planning projects, and the approaches used in AIDS projects promote population control rather than the treatment of people with AIDS. In many African countries, both AIDS control and family planning projects are designed as so-called "vertical" or single-purpose programs that remain outside the broad ("horizontal") basic health services. These programs do not acknowledge that AIDS is a family disease, a disease that affects the health, not just of sexually active adults, but of all family members, directly or indirectly. Although I favor public health and prevention, I have the uneasy feeling that our previous demands for preventive medicine are being turned against us in this case, and that an uncertain prevention is being substituted for treatment. That there is no known cure for AIDS is but a partial explanation because the conditions associated with the syndrome can be treated and some, notably tuberculosis, can be cured.

Third, USAID is giving little assistance to African health services beyond the training of some health workers, and that training is single purpose; for example, laboratory technicians are trained to recognize STDs only, despite the plethora of opportunistic infections associated with AIDS that need diagnosis and treatment. Before 1993, AIDS laboratories did not even screen for tuberculosis, which is highly correlated with HIV positive.

Fourth, initial assistance to STD surveillance was part of the evaluation of intervention projects rather than for the treatment or cure of disease. "Targeted STD surveillance . . . can serve as a proxy for changes in HIV incidence, since few if any projects will be able to demonstrate a direct effect on HIV transmission" (AIDSTECH/Family Health International 1990, 18). This has changed somewhat with the discovery that the presence of untreated STDs accelerates the transmission of HIV, and some aid is now going to the treatment of STDs.

Fifth, USAID assistance in the category "health care financing" revolves around financial planning, which is of interest to the multinational pharmaceutical industry. Assistance is currently directed to the development of a cost model that countries can use to plan transfusion services; the object is to implement cost recovery programs— in other words, fees for blood transfusions and for HIV testing (AIDSTECH/Family Health International 1990:11). So far, aid to HIV surveillance seems to result in recommendations that blood transfusions be reduced to a minimum, rather than to making blood supplies safe.

Finally, having decided that "intravenous drug use plays only a minimal role in HIV transmission" in Africa, USAID (1990:7) says little about contaminated needles and syringes in medical settings. Vachon, Coulaud and Katlama (1985) point out that disposable injection kits, which were first introduced in Africa in the 1970s, are systematically reused in medical practice, even though they cannot be sterilized. Used items are also openly resold: I photographed a large bin of used syringes and needles for sale in a Moroccan market in July 1993. USAID's (1990:40) response is not, in prevailing conditions of scarcity, to supply autoclaves and conventional reusable syringes, but rather to support research on a prefilled injection device that holds a single dose of vaccine or medication in a nonreusable syringe with an attached needle, and on a device that allows only one filling of a syringe designed to be disposable. Scarce foreign exchange will be used to import these devices.

In summary, the main preventive strategy is to persuade sexually active adults to use condoms. USAID purchased 850 million condoms in 1989 and distributed 165 million of them in Africa (Harris 1990). In 1991, USAID obligated $5.2 million to sixteen African countries for condom supply and promotion and other family planning activities. Although Quinn (1990) says condoms confer good protection against HIV infection, there are few data on efficacy in natural as opposed to laboratory settings (Turner, Miller, and Moses 1989, 133). Tropical heat is known to affect rubber, which is biodegradable, so that the shelf life of condoms may be limited. The efficacy of good condoms has also been questioned. Fineberg (1988) showed that condom use is not always a highly effective protection strategy where the prevalence of HIV infection is high among potential partners, as it is in some African cities. In an analysis of one thousand acts of anal intercourse, Fineberg found that full-time condom use cuts the cumulative risk of infection by only 36 percent. In light of these findings, USAID's almost exclusive emphasis on condom supply and promotion calls for a complex explanation.

Conclusion: The Underlying Policy Objectives

The type of assistance the U.S. government is providing to Africa seems to be determined by policy considerations as much as by science, medicine, or public health. The policy considerations concern macroeconomic issues of third world development, and the scientific issues, as described above, appear to be limited to specific experiments in the control of AIDS that may have application in the United States. The macroeconomic issues are not confined to Africa; they include balance of payments deficits and the inability of third world countries to repay bank loans. In response to these problems, the International Monetary Fund (IMF) and the World Bank are promoting structural adjustment programs, which comprise a set of economic reforms that includes currency devaluation, export promotion, import reduction, and the curtailment of government expenditure. Their goal is the repayment of outstanding debts.

Since 1980, IMF and World Bank balance of payments loans have supported economic reform programs in some forty African countries; the minimum condition for these loans is the adoption of specific policies that shape the economic reforms (Loxley 1990:8). In addition to an auction system to determine exchange rates, the IMF and the World Bank require increased domestic currency prices for exports, price liberalization, and increased incentives to the private sector; both agencies treat the food production sector as a "virtual "residual" in the programs of most countries producing agricultural crops for export" (Loxley 1990:15).

Rising levels of unemployment and bread riots are but two indicators of the social damage caused by these reforms. UNICEF has documented the impact of structural adjustment on child health and health services (Cornia, Jolly, and Stewart 1987). For example, currency devaluation reduces individual and government spending power for purchases of life-sustaining necessities (food, clean water, shelter), as well as health care. Export promotion increases workloads, which fall especially heavily on Africa's women farmers, affecting their health and that of their children. Import reduction, particularly in combination with currency devaluation, affects the flow of medical and pharmaceutical supplies and equipment into the many African countries that do not produce their own. The curtailment of government expenditure has more seriously affected health, education, and welfare than other services. The IMF and the World Bank advise most African governments to charge for health services, a burden that falls disproportionately on the poor (see Turshen [forthcoming] for a study of the impact on Zimbabwe). The net result is a decline in both health status and health care in Africa. In the words of a *Lancet* editorial, "there is mounting evidence of deteriorating welfare conditions—e.g., as measured by infant mortality, nutritional status, and educational enrolment—throughout Africa," and "the quality of health services overall has deteriorated . . . "(*Lancet* 1990:885).

Rather than use the AIDS epidemic as an opportunity to redress the underfinancing of African health services, USAID would seem to be pursuing its long-desired program goal of population control. The agency is insisting on the nature of AIDS as an STD, the heterosexual transmission of AIDS in Africa, and the importance of condom use to prevent HIV transmission. Of course condoms also prevent conception. Although USAID projects a 30 to 50 percent increase in child mortality as a result of the epidemic, it expects the population growth rate to decline by only 1 percent, because total fertility is so high in Africa (Harris 1990). USAID concludes, "Not only is this not the time to diminish family planning efforts, but instead such efforts could be redoubled . . . " (Merritt, Lyerly, and Thomas 1988: 127)

The United Nations Conference on Population and Development, held in Cairo in September 1994, made clear the U.S. position on the importance of population control. In fiscal year 1995, the U.S. will devote $600 million to population programs, of which $190 million will be used to support projects run by private organizations and $60 million to purchase contraceptives (*New York Times* September 12, 1994). The *Times* quoted the Rockefeller Foundation, an organization long in the forefront of population activities, as saying that the U.S. is going through a period of reassessment of foreign aid that "involves a reallocation of resources toward population [control] and away from other areas."

Notes

1. It would seem that a small firm, formed in 1970s to respond to the demand for consultants in family planning, expanded in the 1980s to address funding opportunities in AIDS prevention provided by USAID. The question many Africans in governments and universities have about these organizations is how much expertise do they really offer and how much relevant experience do they have in African countries?

2. KAP surveys were initially developed for family planning programs to establish baseline data on contraceptive attitudes and behavior.

3. In 1989, USAID (1990:40,45,62) gave money for field trials and later the purchase of three new commercial rapid blood screening tests developed privately by Dupont, Abbott, and Fujirebo (a Japanese pharmaceutical company). These tests screen pooled blood (i.e. samples are mixed together) and the results cannot be used to advise individuals of their HIV status.

4. I use the term NGO to cover both NGOs and PVOs. According to Green (quoted in Gilson and Sen 1993:5), six types of NGO operate in the health sector--religious organizations, international social welfare groups, local welfare groups, professional associations and unions, nonprofit specialist groups (concerned with occupational health, for example), and nonprofit prepaid health care plans like HMOs. This discussion concerns the northern-based organizations in the first two groups: international church missions and nongovernmental international aid agencies like CARE. I refer to them collectively as NNGOs—northern NGOs operating in the south.

5.   The US Government was not alone in adopting this policy: other northern governments elected to channel funds through their NGOs rather than through multilateral organizations or directly to third world governments. In 1986, an estimated $1 billion is thought to have reached Africa in this way (DeJong 1991:3). As a result the number of NGOs is growing. About one-third of NNGO funds come from their governments (see UNDP 1993: 88-89 for a discussion of funding). Some NNGOs form "partnerships" and fund NGOs in the south, but the UNDP admits that in practice these relationships are far from equal. NGOs are proliferating all over the world.

PART FOUR

Conclusion

14

AIDS: Body, Mind, and History

Shirley Lindenbaum

Introducing his book on epidemic disease in the late 1950's, Arthur Gale suggested that the value of such a volume lay in the "light it throws upon the present because many of the diseases to be discussed have vanished from the English scene or have become trivial"(1959:13). Our confidence about the end of infectious disease as a major public health hazard was shaken by the unexpected emergence of AIDS in the 1980's, even in the industrialized nations. By the 1990's, our security was further undermined by the worldwide emergence of new and resurgent epidemic diseases that, in addition to AIDS, included Legionnaire's disease, Lyme disease, Lassa fever and illness from the Ebola and Marburg viruses. Some of these new and emerging infections are said to be part of the poorly understood "natural cycles" of epidemics, while others are said to reflect the changes that accompany population growth, expanding poverty, urban migration, increasing international travel and changing technology (*Altman, New York Times*, May 10,1994, p.C3).

The contributors to this volume touch upon these combined medical and social themes. The biology, epidemiology, history and social context of infectious diseases now preoccupy scholars worldwide. AIDS, in particular, takes center stage in popular culture (theater, books, film, music, and even humor) as well as in academic research. From 1983 to mid-1991, for example, the MEDLINE database has included more than 200,000 AIDS-related citations from approximately 4000 journals, published in 36 languages from 75 countries (*AIDS and Society* Jan/Feb 1994:1). AIDS may be the most widely discussed disease in the history of medicine.

Giving special attention to AIDS in Africa and the Caribbean, the essays in this volume also illustrate the way in which scholars from different disciplines (in the study of medicine and social life) have begun speaking to each other in an attempt to find a common language. Criticism of the concept of "risk groups," for example, has provided a fruitful terrain for contextualizing epidemiology. In these encounters, many anthropologists have acquired a better appreciation of statistical methods and the way in which science is produced.

In recent years, it has become apparent that AIDS varies widely among neighboring populations and countries, even those with apparently similar demographic profiles. The uneven distribution and spread of the virus is matched by highly uneven patterns of impact. In parts of sub-Saharan Africa, for example, at least as many women as men are infected, in contrast to patterns in Western Europe, Australia and North America. These differences arise not so much from inherent biological differences among individuals and groups, but from differences in patterns of behavior. The AIDS pandemic is no longer viewed as a single phenomenon, for which we might find a simple, universal solution. Instead, different neighborhoods, cities, regions and countries require different intervention strategies (Jonsen and Stryker 1993; Aggleston et al. 1994). Case studies from the Caribbean and Africa thus document the historical and social contexts by which these differences become explicable in order that appropriate interventions and policy decisions can be made.

The worldwide concern for the victims of AIDS, for those who endure the disease as well as for their families and caretakers, also draws our attention to a dimension of the epidemic that increases the suffering—he burden of stigma. The topic of stigma, addressed by many of the authors here, has been widely documented in recent accounts of AIDS in the industrialized democracies (Kirp and Bayer 1992); in the United States in particular (Treichler 1987; Quimby 1992; Padgug and Oppenheimer 1992), as well as in Haiti (Farmer 1992, 1994); Africa (Watney 1988; Packard and Epstein 1992) and elsewhere.

This focus on the moral dimension of the epidemic belongs to a broader discussion of disease and stigmatization in general (Rosenberg 1962; Brandt 1987; Gussow 1989; Rosner and Markowitz 1991). Epidemics, like the diseases that comprise them, are both biological and socio-cultural events. Their material and social profiles are shaped by particular political, economic and cultural circumstances. Epidemics reinforce social boundaries that at other times are less well defined (Lindenbaum 1994).

As many observers have noted, AIDS was first defined as a sexually transmitted disease among marginalized groups, and in the Christian West, quickly became a metaphor for the sin of homosexuality (Gilman 1987; Poirier 1988). When attention moved to other areas of the world and other modes of transmission, a "moral mutation" also occurred, providing us with culturally misleading and judgmental images of the sexual propensities and promiscuity of others. The racist views held about Africans, described above by Lyons and Chirimuuta and Chirimuuta, provide a particularly telling example. In the Caribbean, similar processes were at work as the script for Haitians began to generate images of "squalor, voodoo, and boatloads of 'disease-ridden' or 'economic' refugees" bringing AIDS to the United States (Farmer 1994:340). As a result, the improper identification of Haitians as a "risk group" tarnished a whole community, and placed an additional burden on those suffering from the disease.

The AIDS pandemic has, in effect, given us an opportunity to examine the way we think, talk, and write about people unlike ourselves. AIDS has also emerged at a time when scholars are questioning the manner in which knowledge, power and authority are socially and culturally reproduced in ways that may be opaque to the actors. Our understanding that Western models had come to dominate supposedly universal views of reality has been enhanced by the many contributors to these revelatory discussions. Gays, Haitians, Africans and others now speak for themselves, forcing us to re-evaluate the limits of our knowledge and of legitimate procedures for knowing. These voices of dissent and difference were always present, but the opportunity to reach an outside audience was not as readily available. While AIDS has thus provided the opportunity to further stigmatize certain groups, it has simultaneously brought these alternative voices into a common discussion.

The chapters by Maryinez Lyons and Rosalind and Richard Chirimuuta show that non-Western views of the AIDS pandemic provide a double set of information: indigenous theories of disease causation, as well as a criticism of the potential bias in Western science and Western thought. Placed side by side, Western theories about disease transmission seem no less fantastic than local views on the same topic. While Western commentators have often suggested that bizarre sexual activities and magical practices might provide the key to HIV transmission (Chirimuuta and Chirimuuta above; Farmer 1992:3), local views counter with what might be glibly dismissed as theories of conspiracy. Expressing the thought that some populations provide the fodder for scientific experimentation, or even eradication, the ideas of the sufferers are remarkably uniform, whether they come from Africa, the Caribbean or the United States (Lyons above; Farmer 1992; Lindenbaum 1994).

Similar views have been conveyed in other epidemics and at other times. During the Indian plague in the late nineteenth century, for example, British imagination was fired by a variety of Indian dangers, political, moral, cultural and sanitary. This led to massive state intervention, meddling with caste and religious practices, and a proscription on the free movement of the Indian population. Indians, on the other hand, responded by attacking sanitary inspectors and by concealing plague patients. At the same time, Indian newspapers suggested that the British were systematically poisoning hospital food, the village well, or the municipal water supply. Some reports proposed that the plague did not exist at all, but had been invented to enable government servants to plunder the people, or for doctors to improve their business (Arnold 1987; Chandavarkar 1992). As Arnold comments, the Indian plague provides an "extended commentary on the developing relationship between indigenous elites, subaltern classes and the colonial state" (1987:56), an interpretation that applies well to the participants in the AIDS debate. In the case of AIDS, fears of eradication are not to be lightly dismissed as mere paranoia, given the well publicized reports of some evangelists, politicians and others, that the epidemic is God's judgment on a society that does not live by His rules (Poirier 1988; Showalter 1990; Koop 1991). Moreover, the often-stated belief among minorities in the

United States that AIDS is genocide in the form of germ warfare, or results from lack of attention to an accident in government-sponsored research, reflects the experience of those who live in communities with disproportionately high levels of AIDS, compounded by inadequate health services, low incomes, and rates of infectious disease that interact synergistically with the spread of the HIV virus.

The recent scandals in Japan, France, and elsewhere concerning government distribution of infected blood transfusion products (*Nature* 1988: 331,552; *Science* 1992:258,735), as well as the Tuskegee Syphilis Study in the United States (Brandt 1987:157-8), further remind us that the government is sometimes implicated in killing rather than in saving its citizens. The lesson of AIDS is that competing interpretations and counter histories of the pandemic contain theories of reality from particular vantage points, often based on false perceptions, assumptions and stereotypical views of the behavior and beliefs of others. Racial and ethnic stereotypes color the thinking of each, but dominant groups and the voice of science lends greater authority to one side rather than another. More than a briefing on discrimination, the study of rumors and counter-histories furnishes a warning about the potential routes by which bias may enter into scientific investigation.

The pandemic of AIDS thus provides an opening for many contributors to question the special role of science in the construction of a world culture. Voices from various disciplines, from centers and peripheries, and from dominant and subject positions, are joined in a common discussion about the way science is produced, theories are constructed, and knowledge disseminated. The underbelly of this debate concerns our commitment to the kind of world we are struggling to fashion. The AIDS pandemic is the painful illustration of an international political economy with its cavernous inequalities in economics, health care, disease and suffering.

References

Adebajo, C.O. 1989. "Traditional Practices that are Harmful to Health." Paper Presented at a Meeting of the Inter-African Consultative Expert Group on the Possible Link Between Traditional Practices and the Transmission of HIV, Addis Ababa, May 9-11.

Adegboye, A. 1994. "Health Workers' Attitudes to a Hospitalized AIDS Patient in Ile-Ife, Nigeria: Urgent Need for Intervention [Letter]." *Tropical Doctor.* 24(1):34.

Advisory Group on AIDS. 1986. "Update on AIDS." *South African Medical Journal.* 70:639.

African Rights. 1994. *Rwanda: Death, Despair and Defiance.* London: African Rights.

Aggleston, Peter, Kevin O'Reilly, Gary Slutkin, Peter Davies. 1994. "Risking Everything? Risk Behavior Change and AIDS." *Science.* 265, 341-345.

Ahmed, S.A.; Hamad, E.H.; Kheir, M. 1990. "Sudanese Sexual Behaviour in the Context of Socio-Cultural Norms and the Transmission of HIV." Paper presented at the *IUSSP Seminar on Anthropological Studies Relevant to the Sexual Transmission of HIV.* Sonderborg, Denmark, 19-22 November.

AIDS & Society: International Research and Policy Bulletin. 1990. 1(4):19.

AIDSTECH/Family Health International. 1990. *Semi-Annual Report., 1 October 1989-31 March 1990.* Durham, NC.: AIDSTECH/Family Health International.

Akeroyd, A.V. 1990a. "'Useful' and/or 'Interesting'? Methods for Whom and for What in HIV/AIDS Research in Developing Countries." Based on a Paper for the *Overseas Development Administration Conference, AIDS in Developing Countries: Appropriate Social Research Methods.* Brunel University, Uxbridge.

Akeroyd, A.V. 1990b. "Sociocultural Aspects of AIDS in Africa: Topics, Methods and Some Lacunae." Paper Presented at the *Conference on AIDS in Africa and the Caribbean: The Documentation of an Epidemic.*Columbia University, New York.

Akeroyd, A.V. 1991. "Women, Food Production and Property Rights: Constraints on Women Farmers in Southern Africa," in H. Afshar, ed. *Women, Development and Survival in the Third World.* Pp.139-171. Harlow: Longman.

Akeroyd, A.V. 1994a. "Gender, Race and Ethnicity in Official Statistics: Social Categories and the HIV/AIDS "Numbers Game," in H. Afshar and M. Maynard, eds. *The Dynamics of 'Race' and Gender: Some Feminist Interventions.* Pp. 63-81. London: Taylor & Francis Ltd.

Akeroyd, A.V. 1994b. "HIV/AIDS in Eastern and Southern Africa." *Review of African Political Economy.* 60:173-184.

Akeroyd, A.V. 1994c. "Sex, Social Categories and Silences: Research on HIV/AIDS in Africa." Paper Presented to the Centre for African Studies, University of Liverpool, November 1994.

Aldhous, P.; Tastemain, C. 1987. "Three Physicians Convicted in French 'Blood-Supply Trial.'" [News] *Science.* 258 (5083): 735.

Allen, S. et al. 1989. "Acceptability of Condoms and Spermicides in a Population Based Sample of Urban Rwandan Women." *IV International Conference on AIDS.* Stockholm, Sweden, June 12-16, 1988. Book 1, 349, Abstract 5137.

Altman, Lawrence K. 1992. "Researchers Report Much Grimmer AIDS Outlook: Not Enough Money, Not Enough People, Not Much Hope." *New York Times*. Jun 4 '92.A, 1:2.F.

Altman, Lawrence K. 1994. "Science Times: Infectious Diseases on the Rebound in the U.S., A Report Says." *New York Times*. 10 May, 94: C3.

Alvarez Vazquez, L. and Alvarez La Jonchere, C. 1978. *Cuba: Fecundidad, Diferenciales, Contracepcion y Abortos en Zonas Seleccionadas*. Havana: Instituto de Desarrollo de la Salud.

Amati-Aiah, Edward. 1991. [Of] Makerere University in a Letter to *New Vision*, Sept 5,1991.

Ampofo, E.K. et al. July 1990. "Risk Factors of Vesico-Vaginal Fistula in Maiduguri, Nigeria: a Case Control Study." *Tropical Doctor*. 20(3):138-139.

Anderson, R.M. 1991. "Mathematical Models of the Potential Demographic Impact of AIDS in Africa." *AIDS*. 5 Suppl. (1): 537-544.

Andreani, T.; Le Charpentier, Y.; Brouet J-C. et al. 1983. "Acquired Immunodeficiency with Intestinal Cryptosporidiosis: Possible Transmission by Haitian Whole Blood." *Lancet*. 1(8335): 1187-1191.

Ankrah, E.M., 1991. "AIDS and the Social Side of Health." *Social Science and Medicine*. 32 (9):967-80.

Ankrah, E. M. 1993. "The Impact of HIV/AIDS on the Family and Other Significant Relationships in Africa: The African Clan Revisited." *AIDS Care*. 5(1):5-22.

Anon. 1990. "Structural Adjustment and Health in Africa." *Lancet*. 335 (8694):885-886.

Anon. 1994. "Beauty Who Contaminated 300 Lovers." *New African.*, February, 1994, no. 315: 22.

Appadurai, A. 1991. "Global Ethnoscapes: Notes and Queries for a Transnational Anthropology." in Richard G. Fox (ed.) *Recapturing Anthropology: Working in the Present*. Pp. 191-210. Santa Fe: School of American Research Press.

Aral, S.O. and Holmes, K.K. 1991. "Sexually Transmitted Diseases in the AIDS Era." *Scientific American*. 264(2): 62-69.

Ariyanayagam S. 1991. "Interview with Dr. Jorge Perez." *Cuba Update*. (Summer):23-24.

Arkovitz, M.S.; Manley, M. 1990. "Specialization and Referral Among the N'anga (Traditional Healers) of Zimbabwe." *Tropical Doctor*. 20: 109-110.

Armstrong, A. K. 1987. "Access to Health Care and Family Planning in Swaziland." *Studies in Family Planning*. 18(6):371-382.

Arnold, David 1987. "Touching the Body: Perspectives on the Indian Plague, 1896-1914." in T. Ranger and P. Slack., eds. *Epidemics and Ideas*. p. 203-240. Cambridge: Cambridge University Press.

Auerbach, L.S. 1982. "Childbirth in Tunisia: Implications of a Decision-Making Model." *Social Science and Medicine*. 16: 1499-1506.

Autran, B.; Gorin, I.; Leibowitch, M. et al. 1983. "AIDS in a Haitian Woman with Cardiac Kaposi's Sarcoma and Whipples Disease." *Lancet*. 1(8327): 767-768.

Azicri, M. 1988. *Cuba: Politics, Economics and Society*. London: Pinter Publishers.

Baez, F. 1986. "Braceros Hatianos en la Republica Dominicana." *Instituto Domiicano de Investigaciones Sociales*.

Bagyendera, Hope. 1990. *Weekly Topic*. August 30, 1990.

Barbour, R. S. 1994. "The Impact of Working with People with HIV/AIDS: A Review of the Literature." *Social Science & Medicine*. 39(2):221-232.

Barker , Carol and Meredith Turshen. 1987. "AIDS in Africa." *Revue Of Political Economy*. : 51.

Barnett, T.; Blaikie, P. 1990. "Community Coping Mechanisms in AIDS Affected African Countries: Some Methodological and Conceptual Issues." Revised Version of a Paper Prepared for the *Overseas Development Administration Conference, 'AIDS' in Developing Countries: Appropriate Social Research Methods'*, Brunel University, Uxbridge, 10-11 May 1990.

Barnett, T. and Blaikie, P. M. 1992. *AIDS in Africa: Its Present and Future Impact*. London: Belhaven Press.

Bassett, M.T. and Mhloyi, M. 1991. "Women and AIDS in Zimbabwe: The Making of an Epidemic." *International Journal of Health Services*. 21(1):143-156.

Bayley A.C. 1983. "Aggressive Kaposi's Sarcoma in Zambia." *Lancet*. 1(8390): 1318-1320.

Bayley, A.C. 1990. "Surgical Pathology of HIV Infection: Lessons from Africa." *British Journal of Surgery*. 77(8): 863-868.

Beck, Ann. 1970. *A History of The Brittish Medical Administration of East Africa. 1990-1950*. Cambridge: Harvard University Press.

Beck, D. May 1991. American College of Nurse-Midwives. Personal Communication.

Beers, C. et al. 1988. "AIDS: The Grandmother Burden." in A.F. Fleming et al., eds. *The Global Impact of AIDS*. New York: Liss.

Beeson, D. et al. 1987. "Client-Provider Transactions in Family Planning Clinics." In Robert J. Lapham and George B. Simmons, eds. *Organizing for Effective Family Planning Programs*. Pp. 435-456 Washington, D.C.: National Academy Press.

Belsey, M.A. 1980. "Infertility: Etiology and Natural History." In P.J.Rowe and S.R. Raharinosy-Ramarozaka, eds., *Workshop on the Diagnosis and Treatment of Infertility*, Nairobi, Kenya, 21-22 February 1979. Pp. 11-42. Bath, England: Pitman Press.

Benjamin, M. et al. 1984. *No Free Lunch - Food and Revolution in Cuba Today*. San Francisco: Institute for Food and Development Policy.

Berkley, S.; Maamara, W; Okware, S.I. et al. 1990. "AIDS and HIV Infection in Uganda-- Are More Women Infected than Men?" *AIDS*. 4 (12):1237-1242.

Berkley, S.; Okware, S.I. and Naamara, W. 1989. "Surveillance for AIDS in Uganda." *AIDS*. 3 (2): 79-85.

Berkley, S. F.; Widy-Wirski, B.; Okware, S.; Downing, R.; Linnan, M.J.; White, K.E. and S. Sempala. 1989. "Risk Factors Associated with HIV Infection in Uganda." *The Journal of Infectious Diseases*. 160(1):22-30.

Berlin, E.A. 1985. "Aspects of Fertility Regulation Among the Aguaruna Jívaro of Peru," in Lucile F. Newman, ed., *Women's Medicine: A Cross-Cultural Study of Indigenous Fertility Regulation*. Pp. 125-146. New Brunswick, N.J.: Rutgers University Press.

Berrueta-Clement, John R. et al. 1984. *Changed Lives: The Effects of the Perry Preschool Program on Youths Through the Age 19*. Ysplianti, MI: High Scope Press.

Biggar R.J. 1986a. "The AIDS Problem in Africa. " *Lancet*. 1(8472): 79-83.

Biggar R.J. 1986b. "Possible Nonspecific Associations Between Malaria and HTLV lll/LAV." *New England. Journal Medicine*. 315 (7): 457-458.

Biggar, R.J.; Johnson, B.K.; Oster, G. et al. 1985. "Regional Variations in Prevalence of Antibody Against Human T-Lymphotrophic Virus Types I and III in Kenya, East Africa." *International Journal of Cancer*. 35: 763-767.

Biggar, R.J.; Melbye, M.; Kestens L. et al. 1985. "Seroepidemiology of HTLV-lll Antibodies in a Remote Population of Eastern Zaire." *British Medical Journal*. 290: 808-810.

Birmingham, D. 1989. "Angola Revisited." *Journal of Southern African Studies*. 15(1):1-14.

Bitangaro, Barbara. 1991. "AIDS: Museveni Blames Cultures." *New Vision*. August 10, 1991.

Bitaroho-Kabwa. 1991. AIDS Co-ordinator, Basic Health Services, Fort Portal, quoted in *New Vision.*, 10 Sept 1991.

Blanco, G. 1991. *Concert Against AIDS.* Granma, Feb. 3, 1991.

Bledsoe, C. 1989. "The Cultural Meaning of AIDS and Condoms for Stable Heterosexual Relations in Africa: Recent Evidence from the Local Print Media." Paper presented at the *IUSSP Seminar on Population Policy in Subsaharan Africa: Drawing on Internationl Experience*, Kinshasha, Feb. 27-Mar. 2, Cited in van de Walle q.v.

Bolton, R. and Singer, M.1992. Introduction. Rethinking AIDS and AIDS Prevention: Critical Assesments of the Content and Delivery of Aids Risk-Reduction Messages. *Medical Anthropology.* 14:139-143.

Bond, G.C. and Vincent, J. 1988a. "Field Report on AIDS in Uganda." HIV Center, New York State Psychiatric Institute and Columbia University Presbyterian Hospital. Pp. 47.

Bond, G.C. and Vincent, J. 1988b. "AIDS and Famine in Uganda: The Ethnic Dimension." *Columbia University Seminar on Cultural Pluralism.*, 11 October. Pp. 25.

Bond, G.C. and Vincent, J. 1990. *AIDS and African Economic Development: A Review of the Literature.* Pp. 28.

Bond, G.C. and Vincent, J. 1991a. *Issues Report: HIV/AIDS in African Development. A Report to the United Nations Development Program .(UNDP)*, January 1991. Pp.18.

Bond, G.C. and Vincent, J. 1991b. "Living on the Edge: Structural Adjustment in the Context of AIDS", in H.Bernt Hansen and Michael Twaddle, eds., *Changing Uganda: the Dilemmas of Structural Adjustment and Revolutionary Change.* London: James Currey.

Bond, G.C. and Vincent, J. 1991c. "Women and Children First and Last: AIDS in Uganda." *IUAES* Commission on Women, North American Region, May 30-31.

Bond, G.; A.Z. Rijal and J. Vincent. 1991. "Issues Paper: HIV/AIDS and African Development. A Report to the United Nations Development Program UNDP for Brazzaville Cluster Meeting, March 1991." 18pp.

Bonneux, L.; Van der Stuyft, P.; Taelman H. et al. 1988. "Risk Factors for Infection with Human Immunodeficiency Virus Among European Expatriates in Africa." *British Medical Journal.* 297: 581-584.

Borgdorff, M. M.; Barongo, L. R.; Newell, J.N.; Senkoro, K. P.; Deville, M.; Velema, J. P. and Gabone, R.M.1994. "Sexual Partner Change and Condom Use Among Urban Factory Workers in Northwest Tanzania." *AIDS* . 70(6):378-383.

Brandt, Allan M. 1987. *No Magic Bullet. A Social History of Venereal Disease in the United States Since 1880.* New York: Oxford University Press.

Brown, C. 1982. "Kgatleng Burial Societies." *Botswana Notes and Records.* 14: 80-83.

Browner, C. H. 1985. "Traditional Techniques for Diagnosis, Treatment, and Control of Pregnancy in Cali, Colombia," in Lucile F. Newman. ed., *Women's Medicine: A Cross-Cultural Study of Indigenous Fertility Regulation.* Pp. 99-123. New Brunswick, N.J.: Rutgers University Press.

Brun-Vezinet, F.; Katlama, C.; Roulot, D. 1987. "Lymphadenopathy-Associated Virus Type 2 in AIDS and AIDS-Related Complex: Clinical and Virological Features in Four Patients." *Lancet.* 1(8525): 128-132.

Brunet, J.B.; Chaperon, J.; Gluckman J. C. et al. 1983. "Acquired Immunodeficiency in France."[Letter]*Lancet.*1(8326 Part 1):700-701.

Bundage, J.F. et al. 1990. "Tracking the Spread of the HIV Infection Epidemic." *Journal of Acquired Immunodeficiency Syndrome.*3:1168-1180.

Burke, D.S. et al. 1988. "Measurement of the False Positive Rate in a Screening Program for HIV Infections." *New England Journal of Medicine* .319(15): 961-964.

Buve, A.; Foster, S.; Mbwili, C.; Mungo, E.; Tollenare, N. and Zeko, M. 1994. "Mortality Among Female Nurses in the Face of the AIDS Epidemic: A Pilot Study in Zambia [Letter]." *AIDS*. 8(3):396.

Buwalda, P.; Kruijthoff, D. J.; de Bruyn, M. and Hogewoning, A. 1994. "Evaluation of a Home-Care/Counselling AIDS Programme in Kgatleng District, Botswana." *AIDS Care*. 6(2):153-160.

Bwayo, J.; Plummer, F.; Omari, M.; Mutere, A.; Moses, S.; Ndinya-Achola, J.; Kreis, J. and Velentg, P. 1994. "The Human Immunodeficiency Virus Infection in Long-Distance Truckdrivers in East Africa." *Archives of Internal Medicine*. 154(12):1391-1396.

Bygbjerg L.C. 1983. "AIDS in a Danish Surgeon (Zaire 1976)[Letter]." *Lancet*.1(8330):925.

Bytchenko B. 1986. "The Role of Quality Control of Blood and Blood Products Containment." *WHO-"Working Papers" AlDS-Forschung (AIFO)* 9: 495.

Cabral, A. J. R. 1993. "AIDS in Africa: Can the Hospitals Cope?" *Health Policy and Planning*. 8(2):157-160.

Cabrera, C. 1991. *Reto a la Muerte*. Granma Int., April 7, 1991.

Caldwell ,J.C.; Caldwell P. and P. Quiggin. 1989. "The Social Context of AIDS in Sub-Saharan Africa." *Population and Development Review*. 15(2): 185-234.

Capellan, M.; Reyes, L. 1990. *Estudio Bateyes*. Programa Control de Enfermedades de Transmission Sexual y SIDA (PROCETS). Republica Dominicana: Secretaria de Estado de Salud Publica y Asistencia Social.

Caputo, Robert. 1988. "Uganda, Land Beyond Sorrow." *National Geographic Magazine*.173(8): 468-491.

Carovano, K. 1990. "More than Mothers and Whores: Redefining the AIDS Prevention Needs of Women." *International Journal of Health Services*. 21(1):131-142.

Carr, Raymond 1984. *Puerto Rico: A Colonial Experiment*. New York: Vintage Books, Random House.

Carswell, J. 1988 Impact of AIDS in the Developing World. *British Medical Bulletin* .44 (1):183-202

Castro de Alvarez, V. Holme 1990. "AIDS Prevention Program for Puerto Rican Women." *Puerto Rican Health Science Journal*. 9(1):37-41.

Cates, W. Jr.; Stewart, F.H.; Trussell, J. 1992. "Commentary: The Quest for Women's Prophylactic Methods--Hopes vs Science." *American Journal of Public Health*. 82(11): 1479-1482.

Chao, A.; Bulterys, M.; Musanganire, F.; Habimana, P.; Nawrocki, P.; Taylor, E.; Dushimimana, A. et al. 1994. "Risk Factors Associated with Prevalent HIV-1 Infection Among Pregnant Women in Rwanda." *International Journal of Epidemiology*. 23(2):371-380.

Chandavarkar, Rajnarayan. 1992. "Plague, Panic and Epidemic Politics in India, 1896-1914." in T.Ranger and P.Slack. eds. *Epidemics and Ideas*. p. 203-240. Cambridge: Cambridge University Press.

Chirimuuta R.C.; Chirimuuta R.J. 1989. *AIDS, Africa and Racism*.2nd Ed. London: Free Association Books.

Cleland, J.G. and J.K. Van Ginneken. 1988. "Maternal Education and Child Survival in Developing Countries: the Search for Pathways of Influence." *Social Science and Medicine*. 27(12):1357-1368.

Colebunders, R.; Mann, J.M.; Francis, H.; Bila, K. 1987. "Evaluation of a Clinical Case Definition of Acquired Immunodeficiency Syndrome in Africa." *Lancet*. 1(8531): 492-494.

Colón, H.M.; Robles, R.; Sahai, H. 1991. "HIV Risk and Prior Drug Treatment among Puerto Rican Intravenous Drug Users." *Puerto Rican Health Science Journal.* 10(2): 83-88.

Consortium for Longitudinal Studies. 1983. *As the Twig is Bent: Lasting Effects of Pre-School Programs.* Hillsdale, NJ: Erlbaum.

Cornia, G.A.; Jolly, R. and F. Stewart. 1987. *Adjustment with a Human Face:Protecting the Vulnerable and Promoting Growth.* Oxford: Clarendon Press.

Cosminsky, S. and Scrimshaw, M. 1980. "Medical Pluralism on a Guatemalan Plantation." *Social Science and Medicine* 14B (4):267-278.

Cowell, Alan. 1994. "The Hidden Population Issue: Money." *New York Times.* Sep. 12 '94. A, 6:4.

Crary, D. 1995. "Generation of Rape is Born in Rwanda." *The Guardian.* (London). 11 February, p.13.

Dallabetta, G. et al. 1990. "Vaginal Tightening Agents as Risk Factors for Acquisition of HIV." *VI International Conference on AIDS*, San Francisco California, June 20-24, 1990. Vol. 1, 1990: 268, Abstract No. TH.C.574.

Daniel, M.D.; Letvin, N.L.; Kanki, P.J. et al. 1985. "Isolation of T-Cell Trophic HTLV-Ill-Like Retrovirus from Macaques." *Science.* 228: 1201-1204.

Danziger, R. 1994. "The Social Impact of HIV/AIDS in Developing Countries." *Social Science & Medicine.* 39(7):905-917.

Davidson B. 1978. *Africa in History.* London: Granada Publishing Ltd.

De Cock, K.M. 1984. "AIDS: An Old Disease from Africa?" *British Medical Journal.* 289: 306-308.

De Cock, K. M.; Lucas, S.; Coulibaly, D.; Coulibaly, I.-M. and Soro, B.1993. "Expansion of Surveillance Case Definition for AIDS in Resource-Poor Countries." *Lancet.* 342:437-438.

de Moya, E. 1989. PROCETS. Personal Communication.

De Schryver, A. and A. Meheus. 1990. "Sexually Transmitted Diseases and Migration." Paper presented at the First Migration Medicine Conference. Geneva: 6-9 Februrary 1990.

Decosas, J. and Pedneault, V. 1992. "Women and AIDS in Africa: Demographic Implications for Health Promotion." *Health Policy and Planning.* 7(3):227-233.

Dellicour, D. and Fransen, L. 1994. "Policies and Strategies of the Community." *HIV & AIDS Action.* 4(2):2-4.

DeJong, J. 1991. "Nongovernmental Organizations and Health Delivery in SubSaharan Africa." Working Papers No. 708, Washington, DC: World Bank.

Dixon-Mueller, R. 1993. "The Sexuality Connection in Reproductive Health." *Studies in Family Planning.* 24(5):269-282.

Dixon-Mueller, R. and Wasserheit, J.1991. *The Culture of Silence: Reproductive Tract Infections Among Women in the Third World.* New York: International Women's Health Coalition.

Dr. S. Oware, 1989. Quoted in *New Vision*. Jan 18, 1989.

Dr. Warren Namaara, 1991. Quoted in *New Vision.* 1991.

Dodge, C. P. and P. D. Wiebe, eds. 1985. *Crisis in Uganda, The Breakdown of Health Services.* Oxford: Oxford University Press.

Dondero, T.S. and Curran, J.W. 1991. "Serosurveillance of HIV Infections (Editorial)." *AJPH.* 81:561-62

Dournon, E.; Penalba, C. ; Saimot, A.G.; Wolfe M. et al. 1983. "AIDS in a Haitian Couple in Paris." [Letter] *Lancet.* 1(8332): 1040-1041.

Duh, Samuel V. 1991. *Blacks and Aids: Causes and Origins.* Newbury Park, CA: Sage Publications.

Duncan, M. E.; Tibaux, G.; Pelzer, A.; Mehari, L.; Peuther, J.; Young, H.; Jamil,Y.; Darougar, S.; Piot, P. and Roggen, E. 1994. "A Socioeconomic, Clinical and Serological Study in an African City of Prostitutes and Women Still Married to Their First Husband." *Social Science & Medicine* 39(3):323-333.

Economist Intelligence Unit (EIU).1990. *Uganda. Country Report No. 4.*London: Economist Intelligence Unit.

Eales, L.J.; Nye, K.E.; Pinching, A.J. 1988. "Group-specific component and AIDS: Erroneous data." [Letter] *Lancet.* 1(8591): 936.

Eales, L.-J.; Parkin, J.M.; Pinching, A.J. et al. 1987. "Association of Different Allelic Forms of Group Specific Component with Susceptibility to and Clinical Manifestations of Human Immunodeficiency Virus Infection." *Lancet.* 1(8540): 999-1002.

Edwards, D.; Harper, P.G.; Pain, A.K. 1984. "Kaposi's Sarcoma Associated with AIDS in a Woman from Uganda." [Letter] *Lancet.* 1(8377): 631-632.

Enyodo, Lawrence. [Interview] 1990. Medical Assistant, Kisiizi Hospital. December 15, 1990.

Erickson, Robert J. 1990. "International Behavioral Responses to a Health Hazard: AIDS." *Social Science & Medicine.* 31(9): 951-962.

Eriki, P. 1988. "Antituberculosis Measures for Displaced Persons." *Bull. Int. Union. Tuberc. Lung Dis.* 64(4): 31-32.

Essex, M. and Kanki, P. 1988. "Reply to Kestler et al." *Nature.* 331: 621-622.

Essex, M. and Kanki, P. 1988. "The Origins of the AIDS Virus." *Scientific American.* 259(4): 64-71.

Faas, L. 1991. *Het Nationale AIDSplan van Cuba.* Master's Thesis in Anthropology, University of Amsterdam, The Netherlands.

Farmer, Paul. 1992. *AIDS and Accusation. Haiti and the Geography of Blame.* Berkeley: University of California Press.

Farmer, Paul. 1994. *The Uses of Haiti.* Monroe, ME:Common Courage Press.

Feinsilver, J. 1989. "Cuba as a World Medical Power:The Politics of Symbolism." *Latin American Research Review.* 24 (2): 1-34.

Ferguson J. 1984. "The Laboratory of Racism." *New Scientist.* 103 (Sept. 27 '84): 18-20.

Fernandez Yero, J.L. 1990. "Desarrollo y Perspectivas de la Tecnologia SUMA en el Estudio de Pesquisajes Masivos." Paper presented at *The III National Congress of Hygiene and Epidemiology,* Havana, Cuba, October, 1990.

Figueroa, J.P. 1991. "Is Serious Research Possible in the Caribbean?" *Ethnicity & Disease.* 1(4): 368-378.

Fineberg, H.V. 1988. "Education to Prevent AIDS: Prospects and Obstacles." *Science.* 239:592-596.

Folch-Lyon, E.; De la Macorra, L. and Schearer, S.B. 1981. "Focus Group and Survey Research on Family Planning in Mexico." *Studies in Family Planning.* 12(12):409-432.

Forster, S.J.; Furley, K.E. 1989. "1988 Public Awareness Survey on AIDS and Condoms in Uganda." *AIDS.* 3(3): 147-154.

Foster, S. 1993. "Maize Production, Drought and AIDS in Monze District, Zambia." *Health Policy and Planning.* 8(3):247-254.

Foucault, Michel. 1980. *Power/Knowledge: Selected Interviews and Other Writings, 1972-1977.* New York: Pantheon Books.

Fox, Daniel; Elizabeth Fee., eds. 1992. *AIDS: The Burdens of History.* Berkeley: University of California Press.

Frank, O. 1983. "Infertility in Sub-Saharan Africa." *Center for Policy Studies Working Papers, No. 97.* June, 1983. New York: The Population Council.

Freudenberg, N. 1990. "AIDS Prevention in the U.S.: Lessons from the First Decade." *International Journal of Health Services.* 20(4): 589-599, 1990.

Fryer P. 1984. *Staying Power: The History of Black People in Britain.* Chapter 7, Pluto Press, London.

Fukasawa, M.; Miura, T.; Hasegawa A. et al. 1988. "Sequence of Simian Immunodeficiency Virus from African Green Monkey, A New Member of HIV/SIV Group." *Nature.* 333: 457-461.

Furley, O. and R. A. May. 1989. "Tanzania's Military Intervention in Uganda." Paper Presented at a Conference on Uganda: Structural Adjustment and Regional Change. Roskilde, Denmark September 20-23.

Gale, A.H. 1959. *Epidemic Diseases.* Harmondsworth, Middlesex, UK:Penguin Books Ltd.

Gallin, R.S.; Govindasamy, P. 1993. "Women, Development and Health. Introduction." *Social Science & Medicine.* 37(11): 1283-1284.

Gallo, R.C.; Sliski, A.; Wong-Staal F. 1983. "Origin of T-Cell Leukaemia-Lymphoma Virus." [Letter] *Lancet.* 2(8356): 962-963.

Gallo R.C. 1986. "The First Human Retrovirus." *Scientific American.* 255: 78-88.

Gallo R.C. 1987. "The AIDS Virus." *Scientific American.* 256(1): 39-48.

Garcia, Rudy. [Interview with Dr. Irene Impelizzeri]. *Noticias del Mundo.*

Garris, I. 1989. "The Wave-Like Progression of AIDS in the Dominican Republic." *PROCETS, Republica Dominicana.*

Garris, I.; Rodriquez, E.M.; De Moya, E.A.; Guerrero, E. et al. 1991. "AIDS Heterosexual Predominance in the Dominican Republic." *Journal of Acquired Immune Deficiency Syndromes.* 4(12): 1173-1178.

Geertz, Clifford. 1983. *Local Knowledge: Further Essays in Interpretive Anthropology.* New York: Basic Books.

Gestin, E.L. 1987. "Social and Community Interventions." *Annual Review of Psychology.* 38:427-60.

Gilks, C. 1991. "AIDS , Monkeys and Malaria". *Nature.* 354: 262.

Gilman, Sander L. 1987. "IDS and Syphilis: The Iconography of Disease." *October.* 43:87-108.

Gilpin, M. 1989. "Cuba: On the Road to a Family Medicine Nation." *Family Medicine.* 21(6): p.409, Oct-Nov. 1989.

Gilson, L. and Sen, P.D. 1993. "Assessing the Potential of Health Sector NGOs: Policy Options." in *Report of the Workshop on the Public/Private Mix for Health Care in Developing Countries*, London: London School of Hygiene and Tropical Medicine.

Good, C. 1988. "Traditional Healers and AIDS Management." in N. Miller & R.C. Rockwell, eds., *AIDS in Africa: The Social and Policy Impact.* Pp.97-113. Leviston/Queenstown: Edwin Mellen Press.

Goodgame, R.W. 1990. "AIDS in Uganda: Clinical and Social Features." *New England Journal of Medicine.* 323(6): 383-389.

Gordon, D. 1991. "Female Circumcision and Genital Operations in Egypt and the Sudan: A Dilemma for Medical Anthropology." *Medical Anthropology Quarterly.* 5(1)1991:3-23.

Gordon, G.; Klouda, T. 1989. *Preventing a Crisis: AIDS and Family Planning Work.* London: Macmillan (for the IPPF).

Gottlieb, Benjamin H. 1983. "Social Support as a Focus for Integrative Research in Psychology." *American Psychologist.* 38(3): 278-287.

Gottlieb, M.S.; Shanker, H.M.; Fan P.T. et al. 1981. "Pneumocystis Pneumonia - Los Angeles." *MMWR.* 30(21): 250-251.

Green, E. C., Dokwe, B. and Dupree, J.D. 1995. "The Experience of an AIDS Prevention Program Focused on South African Traditional Healers." *Social Science & Medicine.* 40(4):505-515.

Green, E. C., Jurg, A. and Dgede, A. 1993. "Sexually Transmitted Diseases, AIDS and Traditional Healers in Mozambique." *Medical Anthropology.* 15(3):261-281.

Green, E.C. and Makhubu, L. 1984. "Traditional Healers in Swaziland: Toward Improved Cooperation Between the Traditional and Modern Health Sectors." *Social Science and Medicine* 18(12):1071-1079.

Grundy, P.H. et al. 1980. "The Distribution and Supply of Cuban Medical Personnel in Third World Countries." *American Journal of Public Health.* 70:717-719.

du Guerny, J. and Sjöberg, E. 1993. "Inter-Relationship Between Gender Relations and the HIV/AIDS Epidemic: Some Possible Considerations for Policies and Programmes." *AIDS.* 7:1027-1034.

Guerrero, E.; Garris, I.; Koenig, G. 1987. *Seroprevalencia del HIV en Obreros Haitiano Migrantes a Dominicana.* Santo Domingo, Ministerio de Salud Publica.

Gussow, Zachary. 1989.*Leprosy, Racism, and Public Health. Social Policy in Chronic Disease Control.* Boulder: Westview Press Inc.

Hamblin, J. and Reid, E. 1991. "Women, the HIV Epidemic and Human Rights: A Tragic Imperative." Paper Prepared for the *International Workshop on "AIDS: A Question of Rights and Humanity, International Court of Justice,*The Hague, May 1991.

Hamilton D. 1986. *The Monkey Gland Affair.* London: Chatto and Windus.

Hansen, K. T. 1994. "Dealing with Used Clothing: Salaula and the Construction of Identity in Zambia's 3rd Republic." *Public Culture.* 6(3):503-523.

Harris, Jeffrey R. 1990. "Statement to Thirty-third Annual Meeting of the African Studies Association," Baltimore, MD. Panel on AIDS: Current State of the Epidemic and Treatments, 3 November.

Hatcher, R.A. et al. 1994. *Contraceptive Technology: International Edition.* Atlanta, GA: Printed Matter, Inc.

Heggenhougen, H.K. 1980. "Bomohs, Doctors and Sinsehs - Medical Pluralism in Malaysia." *Social Science and Medicine.* 14B(4):235-244.

Heise, L. L. and Elias, C. 1995. "Transforming AIDS Prevention to Meet Women's Needs: A Focus on Developing Countries." *Social Science & Medicine.* 40(7):931-943.

Heise, L.L.; Raikes, A.; Watts, C. H.; and Zwi, A.B. 1994. "Violence Against Women: A Neglected Public Health Issue in Less Developed Countries." *Social Science & Medicine.* 39(9):1165-1179.

Herdt, G. and Lindenbaum, S. eds. 1992. *The Time of AIDS: Social Analysis, Theory, and Method.* Newbury Park, CA: Sage Publications.

Hirsch, V.M.; Olmstead, R.A.; Murphey-Corb M. et al. 1989. "An African Primate Ientivirus (SIVsm) Closely Related to HIV-2." *Nature.* 339: 389-392.

Hollerbach, P. and Diaz Briquets, S. 1983. *Fertility Determinants in Cuba.* Washington D.C.: National Academy Press.

Holmberg, S.D. 1996. "The Estimated Prevalence and Incidence of HIV 96 Large US Metropolitan Areas." *American Journal of Public Health.* 86(5): 642-654.

Holmes, K.K. et al. , eds. 1984. *Sexually Transmitted Diseases.* New York: McGraw Hill.

Hooper, E., 1987 "AIDS in Uganda." *African Affairs.* 86.

Hooper, E. and L. Pirouet. 1989. *Uganda.* Minority Rights Group Report No. 66. London.

Hrdy, D.B. 1987. "Cultural Practices Contributing to the Transmission of Human Immunodeficiency Virus in Africa. [Review]. *Reviews of Infectious Diseases.* 9(6): 1109-1119.

Hubert, A. 1990. "Applying Anthropology to the Epidemiology of Cancer." *Anthropology Today.* 6(5): 16-18.

Hudson, C.P. et. al, 1988a. "Risk Factors for the Spread of AIDS in Rural Africa: Evidence from a Comparative Seroepidemiological Survey of AIDS, Hepatitis B and Syphilis in Southwestern Uganda." *AIDS.* 2:255-260.

Hudson, C. P. & Hennis, P. Katarha et al. 1988. "HIV, Hepatitis B and Syphilis in Southwestern Uganda: Comparative Seroepidemiologicals Survey of Risk Factors in the Spread of AIDS in Rural Africa." *AIDS.* 2:255-260.

Hunsmann, G. 1990. *Monkey Business.* Interview on Channel 4 Television, London 23.05 hours G.M.T, 22/1/90.

Hunte, P.A. 1985. Genous Methods of Fertility Regulation in Afghanistan," in Lucile F. Newman, ed., *Women's Medicine: A Cross-Cultural Study of Indigenous Fertility Regulation.* Pp. 43-75. New Brunswick, N.J.: Rutgers University Press.

Hunter, Susan 1990a. "Orphans as a Window on the AIDS Epidemic in Sub-Saharan Africa: Initial Results and Implications of a Study in Uganda."*Social Science & Medicine.* 31(6):681-690.

Hunter, Susan. 1990b. "An Update of the Orphan Situation in Uganda." Paper presented at the *Conference on AIDS: Community Coping Mechanism in the Face of Exceptional Demographic Change.,* Kampala 20.

Hunter, D. J.; Maggwa, B.N.; Mati, J. K. G.; Tukei, P. M.; and Mbugwa, S. 1994. "Sexual; Behaviour, Sexually Transmitted Diseases, Male Circumcision and Risk of HIV-Infection Among Women in Nairobi." *AIDS.* 8(1):93-99.

Huston, Perdita. 1978. *Message From the Village.* New York: The Epoch B Foundation.

Ingstad, B. 1990. "The Cultural Construction of AIDS and its Consequences for Prevention in Botswana." *Medical Anthropology Quarterly* (n.s.) 4(1):28-40.

Interview with Dr. I.S.,1990. 13 Dec 1990.

Interview of Nabbi M, Kyotera, Rakai 1990. On Jan 24, 1991.

Jaffre, Y. and Prual, A. 1994. "Midwives in Niger: An Uncomfortable Position Between Social Behaviours and Health Care Constraints." *Social Science & Medicine.* 38(8):1069-1073.

Jagwe, J.G.M. 1986. *Progress Report on AIDS in Uganda.* The Panos Institute, London.

Janzen, J.M. 1978. *The Quest for Therapy: Medical Pluralism in Lower Zaire.* Berkeley: University of California Press.

Jochelson, K.; Mothibeti, M.; and Leger, J.-P. 1991. "Human Immunodeficiency Virus and Migrant Labor in South Africa." *International Journal of Health Services.* 21(1):157-173.

Johnson, D.L. and Breckenridge, J. 1982. "The Houston Parent-Child Development Center and the Primary Prevention of Behavior Problems in Young Children." *American Journal of Community Psychology.* 10:305-316.

Johnson, D.L. and Walker. 1985. "The Primary Prevention of Behavior Problems in Mexican-American Children."Presented at Social Research and Child Development. Toronto.

Jones P. 1985. "AIDS. The African Connection?" *British Medical Journal:* 290:932.

Jonsen, Albert R. and Jeff Stryker. eds. 1993. *The Social Impact of AIDS in the United States.* National Academy Press, Washington, D.C.

Jordan, Theresa J. et al. 1985. "Long-Term Effects of Early Enrichment: A 20 Year perspective on Persistence and Change. Special Issue: Children's Environments." *American Journal of Community Psychology.* 13(4): 393-415.

Kadura, Godfrey , Enoch Mwesigwe and Alice Nambi. 1990. A Preliminary Report on a Needs Assesment Study of Raki and Masaka Districts with Particular References to the Socio-Economic Impact of the AIDS Epidemic. NS.

Kaijage, F.J. 1993. "AIDS Control and the Burden of History in Northwestern Tanzania." *Population and Environment* 14(3):279-300.

Kalibala, S. and Kaleeba, N. 1989. "AIDS and Community-Based Care in Uganda: The AIDS Support Organisation, TASO." *AIDS Care* 1(2): 173-175.

Kalibbala, Vincent. 1991. Maska reporter for *New Vision.* May 29, 1991.

Kanki, P.J.; Alroy, J.; Essex M. 1985. "Isolation of T-Lymphotropic Retrovirus Related to HTLVIII/LAV from Wild Caught African Green Monkeys." *Science.* 230: 951-954.

Katner, H.P. and Pankey, G.A. 1987." Evidence for a Euro-American Origin of Human Immunodeficiency Virus." *J. National Medical Association.* 79: 1068-1072.

Katonbozi, Reverend Canon [Interview]. 1990. At Kiziiski Hospital,Kabale District. Dec. 15, 1990.

Kazibwe, Leonard. [Interview]. 1991. AIDS Counsellor at Kitovu Hospital, Maska Jan. 9, 1991.

Keogh, P., Allen, S.; Almedal, C. and Temahagili, B. 1994. "The Social Impact of HIV Infection on Women in Kigali, Rwanda: A Prospective Study'." *Social Science & Medicine.* 38(8):1047-1053.

Kerns, V. 1989. *Women and the Ancestors: Black Carib Kinship and Ritual.* Urbana and Chicago: University of Illinois Press, 1989.

Kestler, H.W.; Li, Y.; Naidu, Y.M. et al. 1988. "Comparison of Simian Immunodeficiency Virus Isolates." *Nature.* 331: 619-621.

King, M.B. 1989. "AIDS on the Death Certificate: The Final Stigma." *British Medical Journal.* 298(6675):734-736.

Kirp,David.L. and Ronald Bayer, eds. 1992: *AIDS in the Industralized Democracies: Passions, Politics, and Policies.* Rutgers University Press, N.J.

Kisekka, M. N. 1990. "AIDS in Uganda as a Gender Issue." *Women & Therapy.* 10(3):35-53.

Kloos, H. et al. 1987. "Illness and Health Behavior in Addis Ababa and Rural Central Ethiopia." *Social Science and Medicine.* 25(9):1003-1019.

Koch-Weiser D.; Vanderschmidt, H., eds. 1989. *The Heterosexual Transmission of AIDS in Africa.* Cambridge, MA: Abt Books.

Kohi, T. W. and Horrocks, M.J. 1994. "The Knowledge, Attitudes and Perceived Support of Tanzanian Nurses When Caring for Patients with AIDS." *International Journal of Nursing Studies.* 31(1):77-86.

Konde-Lule, J.K. and Berkley, S.F. and R. Downing. 1989. "Knowledge, Attitudes and Practices Concerning AIDS in Ugandans." *AIDS.* 3(8): 513-518.

Konotey-Ahulu , F.I.D. 1987. "Clinical Epidemiology, not Seroepidemiology, is the Answer to Africa's AIDS Problem." *British Medical Journal.* 294: 1593-1594.

Konotey-Ahulu , F.I.D [Anonymous]. 1987. "Group Specific Component and HIV infection." *Lancet.* 1(8544): 1267-9.

Konotey-Ahulu , F.I.D. 1989. "An African on AIDS in Africa. The AIDS Letter." *Royal Society of Medicine* 11: 1-3.

Koop, C.E. 1991. *Koop. Memoirs of America's Family Doctor.* New York: Random House.

Kreniske, J. 1987. "Leadership in Barrio Ingenio: Acting on a Geopolitical Stage." Presented to Columbia University Seminar on Cultural Pluralism, November.

Kreniske, J. 1988. "AIDS Transmission in the Caribbean." Proceedings, Hunter College Conference on AIDS and Anthropology, City University, New York.

Kuhn, Thomas. 1970. *The Structure of Scientific Revolutions.* 2nd. Ed. Chicago: University of Chicago Press.

Kyarisiima, Mary [Interview]. Kabale. Dec. 17, 1990.

La Cancella, V. de. 1989. "Minority AIDS Prevention: Moving Beyond Cultural Perspectives Towards Sociopolitical Empowerment." *AIDS Education and Prevention.* 1(2): 141-153.

Larson, A. 1989. "Social Context of Human Immunodeficiency Virus Transmission in Africa: Historical and Cultural Bases of East and Central African Sexual Relations." *Reviews of Infectious Diseases.* 11(5):716-731.

Lazar, I.; Darlington, R. 1982. "Lasting Effects of Early Education. A Report from the Consortium for Longitudinal Studies." *Monographs in Social Research and Child Development.* 47(2-3): 1-151.

Lewis, G.K. 1963. *Puerto Rico: Freedom and Power in the Caribbean.* New York : Monthly Review Press.

Lie, G. and Biswalo, P.M. 1994. "Perceptions of the Appropriate HIV/AIDS Counselling in Arusha and Kilimanjaro Regions of Tanzania: Implications for Hospital Counselling." *AIDS Care* 6(2):139-151.

Lindenbaum, S. 1987. "Anthropological Perspectives." In *Comparative Perspectives on AIDS: Proceedings from the Hunter College Conference- Perspectives on AIDS: A Dialogue Between Social Scientists and Health Professionals.* December 15, 1987, pp. 55-62.

Lindenbaum, Shirley. 1994. "Images of Catastrophe: The Making of an Epidemic." in Merrill Singer, Robert Carlson and Steve Koester (eds). *The Political Economy of AIDS.* Baywood Publishing Co. (In Press).

Low, S.M. and Newman, B.C. 1985 "Indigenous Fertility Regulating Methods in Costa Rica." In Lucile F. Newman ed.. *Women's Medicine: A Cross-Cultural Study of Indigenous Fertility Regulation.* Pp.147-160. New Brunswick, N.J.: Rutgers University Press.

Loxley, J. 1990. "Structural Adjustment in Africa: Reflections on Ghana and Zambia." *Review of African Political Economy.* 47:8-27.

Lyons, Maryinez. 1985. "From Death Camps to Cordon Sanitaire: The Development of Sleeping Sickness Policy in the Uele District in the Belgian Congo, 1903-1911." *Journal of African History.* 26: 69-91.

Lyons, Maryinez. 1988a. "Sleeping Sickness, Colonial Medicine and Imperialism: Some Connections in the Belgian Congo." in R.M. Maclead and M. Lewis., eds., *Disease, Medicine, and Empire.* London: Tavistock.

Lyons, Maryinez. 1988b. "Sleeping Sickness, Policy and Public Health in the Early Belgian Congo." in D. Arnold., ed., *Medicine and Empire.* Manchester: Manchester University Press.

Lyons, Maryinez. 1992. *The Colonial Disease: A Social History of Sleeping Sickness in Northern Zaire, 1900-1940.* New York: Cambridge University Press.

MacGaffey, J. 1986. "Women and Class Formation in a Dependent Economy: Kisangani Entrepreneurs." in C. Robertson & I. Berger, eds. *Women and Class in Africa.* Pp. 161-177. New York: Africana Publishing Company.

Maldonado, N. 1990. "Latinas and HIV/AIDS." *SIECUS Report.* December 1990/January 1991:11-15.

Mann, J. 1987. "AIDS in Africa." *New Scientist.* 113 (Mar. 26 '87):40-43.

Manuel, L. 1987. "El Caso Sandra." *Somos Jovenes:* September, 1987.

Marshall, J.F. 1973. "Fertility Regulating Methods: Cultural Acceptability for Potential Adopters," in G.W. Duncan et al. *Fertility Control Methods: Strategies for Introduction.* Pp. 125-132. New York: AcademicPress.

Martinez, A. and Torres, R. 1990. "Epidemiologists at the Santiago de las Vegas Sanatorium." Personal Communication, October.

Massabot, E.R. 1986. National Director of Health Statistics, Personal Communication.

Massabot, E. Rios and A. Tejeiro. 1987. Perfiles de Salud. *Rev. Cub. de Medicina General Integral,* Suplemento.

Mathiot, C.C.; Lepage, C.; Choaib, E.; Georges-Courbert, M-C. & Georges, A.J. 1990. "HIV Seroprevalence and Male to Female Ratio in Central Africa. [Correspondence]." *Lancet.* 375(8690):672.

Mays, V.M.; Cochran, S.D. 1988. "Issues in the Perception of AIDS Risk and Risk Education Activities by Black and Hispanic/Latino Women." *American Psychologist.* 43(11): 949-957.

McFalls, J.A. and McFalls, M.H. 1984. *Disease and Fertility.* New York: Academic Press.

McGrath, J. W.; Ankrah, E. M.; Schumann, D.A.; Nkumbi, S. and Lubega, M. 1993. "AIDS and the Urban Family: Its Impact in Kampala, Uganda." *AIDS Care.* 5(1):55-70.

McGrath, J. W.; Schumann, D.A.; Pearson-Marks, J.; Rwabukwali, C.B.; Mukasa, R.; Namande, B. and Nakayiwa, S. 1992. "Cultural Determinants of Sexual Risk Behavior for AIDS Among Baganda Women." *Medical Anthropology Quarterly.* 6(2):153-161.

McIvor, C. 1994. "Life on the Streets of Harare." *New African.* No.322(September):27.

McKinley, James C. 1996. "A Ray of Light in Africa's Struggle with AIDS." *New York Times.* Apr 7 '96: 1, 1:2.

Mernissi, F. "Obstacles to Family Planning Practice in Urban Morocco." *Studies in Family Planning.* 6(12)1975:418-425.

Merritt, G., W. Lyerly, and J. Thomas. 1988. "The HIV/AIDS Pandemic inAfrica: Issues of Donor Strategy," in N. Miller and R.C. Rockwell, ed., *AIDS in Africa: The Social and Policy Impact.* Pp. 115-129. Lewiston, N.Y.: The Edwin Mellen Press.

Micklin, M.; Sly, D. 1988. "International Population Movements and AIDS: Patterns, Consequences, and Policy Implications," in Fleming et al. pp. 67-77. *The Global Impact of Aids.*

Millan, Juan C. 1988. Personal Communication.

MINSAP. 1969. *Diez Años de Revolucion en Salud Publica.* Editorial Ciencias Sociales, La Habana.

MINSAP. 1970. *Organizacion del Sistema Unico de Salud.* Havana: MINSAP.

MINSAP. 1988. Cuba: 25 Años de Cooperación Médica. Havana: MINSAP.

MINSAP. 1989. *Programa de Control del SIDA, Cronologia l983-l989.* Havana: MINSAP.

MINSAP. 1990a. *Annual Report, l989.* Ministry of Public Health, Havana: MINSAP.

MINSAP. 1990b. Programa de Control del SIDA. *Informe Resumen Hasta el l6 de Enero,* 1990. Unpublished report, MINSAP: Havana.

Mintz, Sidney. 1960. *Worker in the Cane: A Puerto Rican Life History.* New Haven: Yale University Press.

MMWR. 1982. "Opportunistic Infections and Kaposi's Sarcoma among Haitians in the United States." 31:353-354, 360-361.

MMWR. 1987a. 36(5-6): 1-20.

MMWR. 1987b. 36(15): 35-155.

MMWR. 1988. 37(20): 37.

Molyneaux, J.W. et al. 1990. "Correlates of Contraceptive Method Choice in Indonesia." Population Studies in Sri Lanka and Indonesia Based on the *1987 Sri Lankan Demographic and Health Survey and the 1987 National Indonesian Contraceptive Prevalence Survey. The Population Council and Demographic and Health Surveys, Institute for Resource Development, Demographic and Health Surveys Further Analysis Series, No. 2, March 1990.*

Moscoso Puello, F.E. 1981. *La Novela de la Caña.* Santo Domingo, Republica Dominicana: Editora de Santo Domingo.

Moses, S. and F. A. Plummer. 1994. "Health Education, Counselling and the Underlying Causes of the HIV Epidemic in Sub-Saharan Africa." *AIDS Care.* 6(2):123-   127.

Moss A.R. 1988. "Epidemiology of AIDS in Developed Countries." *British Medical Bulletin.* 44(1): 58.

Moya-Pons, Frank. 1986. *El Batey: Estudio Socioeconimico de los Bateyes del Consejo Estatal del Azucar.* Santo Domingo, Dominica Republica: Fondo Para El Avance de Las Ciencias Sociales.

Mulder C. 1988a. "A Case of Mistaken Non-Identity." *Nature.* 331:562-563.

Mulder C. 1988b. "Human Virus not from Monkeys." *Nature.* 333:396.

Muller, D. and   N. Abbas. 1990. "Risk Factors: Cofactors in Heterosexual AIDS Transmission in Uganda." In Ronald E. Watson ed.. *Cofactors in HIV-1 Infection and AIDS.* Boca Baton: CRC press.

Mulwindwa, E. 1990. "Makerere." *Weekly Topic.* December 16, 1990.

Muniz, Jose Gutierrez et al. 1984. "The Recent Worldwide Economic Crisis and the Welfare of Children: The Case of Cuba." *World Development.* 12: 247-260.

Munodawafa, D.; Bower, D. A.; and Webb, A. A. 1993. "Perceived Vulnerability to HIV/AIDS in the US and Zimbabwe." *International Nursing Review.* 40(1):13-16, 24.

Museveni [President], 1990.Reported in *New Vision.* December 3, 1990.

Muzio, V. and Galban Garcia, E. 1990. "Report on the Situation of Hepatitis B in Cuban and Vaccine Research." Paper Presented at the III National Congress of Hygiene and Epidemiology, Havana, Cuba, October, l990.

Mwale, G. and P. Burnard. 1992. *Women and AIDS in Rural Africa: Rural Women's Views of AIDS in Zambia.* Aldershot: Avebury.

National Academy of Sciences (Institute of Medicine). 1986. *Mobilizing Against AIDS:The Unfinished Story of a Virus.* Eve K. Nichols, writer. Cambridge, Mass.: Harvard University Press.

National Research Council. 1989. *AIDS Sexual Behavior and IV Drug Use.* Washington, DC: National Academy Press.

Neequaye, A.R.; Neequaye, J.; Mingle J.A. et al. 1986. "Preponderance of Females with AIDS in Ghana." *Lancet.* 2(8513): 978.

New Scientist. [Editorial.] 1987. "Evidence for Origin is Weak." *New Scientist.* 118 (15):27.

New Vision. 1987. "[Letter] to the Editor.," Sept. 1987.

New Vision (Kampala, Uganda). 1990. July 13, 1990.

New Vision (Kampala, Uganda). 1990. November 5, 1990

New Vision(Kampala, Uganda). 1990. " [Letter] to the Editor." December 14, 1990.

New Vision (Kampala, Uganda). 1991. June 26, 1991.

News: 1990. "Africa: Nursing is on the Agenda of AIDS Conference.", *International Nursing Review.,* 37(4): 291.

Newman, L.F. 1985. "Context Variables in Fertility Regulation," in Lucile F. Newman, ed., *Women's Medicine: A Cross-Cultural Study of Indigenous Fertility Regulation*. Pp. 179-191. New Brunswick, N.J.:Rutgers University Press.

N'Galy, B.; Ryder, R.W.; Bila, K. et al. 1988. "Human Immuno-Deficiency Virus Infection Among Employees in an African Hospital." *The New England Journal of Medicine*. 319(17):1123-1127.

Ngin, C.S. 1985. "Indigenous Fertility Regulating Methods Among Two Chinese Communities in Malaysia." in Lucile F. Newman, ed., *Women's Medicine: A Cross-Cultural Study of Indigenous Fertility Regulation*. Pp. 125-141. New Brunswick, N.J.: Rutgers University Press.

Nkowane, A. M. 1993. "Breaking the Silence: The Need for Counselling of HIV/AIDS Patients." *International Nursing Review*. 40(1):17-20, 24.

Noireau, F. 1987. "HIV Transmission from Monkey to Man." *Lancet*. 1(8548): 1498-1499.

North, B.B. 1990. "Effectiveness of Vaginal Contraceptives in Prevention of Sexually Transmitted Diseases." in Nancy J. Alexander et al., ed., *Heterosexual Transmission of AIDS*. Pp. 273-290. New York: WileyLiss.

Nunn, P.; McAdam K.P. 1988. "AIDS in Africa." *Medicine International*. September: 2357-60.

Nunn, A. J.; Kengeya-Kayondo, J. F.; Malamba, S.; Seeley, J. A.; and Mulder, D. 1994. "Risk Factors for HIV-1 Infection in Adults in a Rural Ugandan Community: A Population Study." *AIDS*. 8(1):81-86.

Nzilambi, N.; De Cock, K.; Forthal D.N. et al. 1988. "The Prevalence of Infection with Immunodeficiency Virus over a 10 year Period in Rural Zaire." *New England Journal of Medicine*. 318(5): 276-279.

Obbo, C. 1991a. "Some Social Issues Arising from the HIV Epidemic in Uganda." Paper Presented at the HIV Center for Clinical and Behavioral Studies, Columbia Prebyterian Medical Center, March 28.

Obbo, C. 1991b. "Reflections on the AIDS Orphans in Uganda, Dossier." *The Courier*. No.126:55-56.

Obbo, C. 1993a. "HIV Transmission: Men are the Solution." *Population and Environment*. 14(3):211-243.

Obbo, C. 1993b. "HIV Transmission Through Social and Geographical Networks in Uganda." *Social Science & Medicine*. 36(7):949-955.

Okojie, C. E. E. 1994. "Gender Inequalities of Health in the Third World." *Social Science & Medicine*. 39(9):1237-1247.

Okware, S.I. 1987. "Towards a National AIDS-Control Program in Uganda." *Western Journal of Medicine*. 147(6): 726-729.

Olowa-Freers. 1990. Cited in Barnett, P.and Blaikie, P. 1990.

O'Malley, P.ed. 1989. *The Aids Epidemic: Private Rights and the Public Interest*. Beacon Press: Boston.

Orubuloye, I.O.; Caldwell, J.C. and Caldwell, P. 1990. "Sexual Networking and the Risk of AIDS in Southwest Nigeria." Paper Delivered at the IUSSP Seminar on Anthropological Studies Relevant to the Sexual Transmission of HIV. Sonderborg, Denmark, 19-22 November 1990.

Orubuloye, I.O.; Caldwell, J. C.; and Caldwell, P. 1993. "African Women's Control over Their Sexuality in an Era of AIDS." *Social Science & Medicine*. 37(7):859-872.

de la Osa, J.A. 1991. "Reportados en lo Que Va de Ano 80 Casos de Portadores del SIDA." *Granma*. May 24, 1991.

Ososanya, O. O. and Brieger, W. R. 1994. "Rural-Urban Mobility in Southwestern Nigeria: Implications for HIV/AIDS Transmission from Rural to Urban Communities." *Health Education Research.* 9(4):507-518.

Owore, D.A. 1990. "Kampala." *New Vision.* December, 1990.

Packard, R.M. 1989. "Epidemiologists, Social Scientists, and the Structure of Medical Research on AIDS in Africa." *Working Papers in African Studies.*, no. 137. Boston: Boston University, African Studies Center.

Packard, Randall M. and Paul Epstein. 1992. "Medical Research on AIDS in Africa: A Historical Perspective." Cited in Padgug, Robert A. and Gerald M. Oppenheimer . "Riding the Tiger: AIDS and the Gay Community", in Elizabeth Fee and Daniel Fox. (eds). *AIDS: The Making of A Chronic Disease.* p. 346-376. Berkeley: University of California Press.

Padgug, Robert A. and Gerald M. Oppenheimer. 1992. "Riding the Tiger : AIDS and the Gay Community." In Elizabeth Fee and Daniel Fox., eds. *AIDS: The Making of a Chronic Disease.* p. 346-376. Berkeley: University of California Press.

Patton, C. 1990. *Inventing AIDS.* NY: Routledge.

Pearson, M. 1988. "What Does Distance Matter? Leprsoy Control in West Nepal." *Social Sciences and Medicine.* 26: 25-36.

Pela, A.O. & Platt, J.J. 1989. "AIDS in Africa: Emerging Trends." *Social Science and Medicine.* 28(1):1-8.

Peña, R. Torres.et al. 1990. "Situacion del SIDA y la Infeccion por VIH en Cuba". Paper Presented at the III National Congress of Hygiene and Epidemiology, Havana, Cuba, October, l990.

Peterman, T.A. 1990. "Facilitators of HIV Transmission During Sexual Contact." in Nancy J. Alexander et al. (eds)., *Heterosexual Transmission of AIDS.* Pp. 55-68. New York: Wiley-Liss.

Pichenik, A.E.; Spira, T.J.; Elie, R.; et al. 1985. "Prevalence of HTLV/LAV Antibodies Among Haitians." *New England Journal of Medicine.* 312 (26):1705.

Pickering, H.; Todd, J.; Dunn, D.; Pepin, J. and Wilkins, A. 1992. "Prostitutes and Their Clients: a Gambian Survey." *Social Science & Medicine.* 34(1):75-88.

Pierson, Donald E. 1984. "A School-Based Program from Infancy to Kindergarten for Children and Their Parents." *Personnel and Guidance Journal.* 62(8):448-455.

Piot, P. & Carael, M. 1988a. "Epidemiological and Sociological Aspects of HIV Infection in Developing Countries." *British Medical Bulletin.* 44(1):66-88.

Piot, P. & Carael, M. 1988b. AIDS and HIV Infection: The Wider Perspective." *British Medical Bulletin.* 44(1): 4.

Poirier,Richard. 1988. "AIDS and Traditions of Homophobia." *Social Research.* 55:3:461-476.

Powell, T.J. 1985. "Improving the Effectiveness of Self-Help." *Social Policy.* 16:22-29.

Pramualratana, Anthony, Chai Podhisita, Uraiwan Kanungsukkasem et al. 1994. "The Social Context of Condom Use in Low-Priced Brothels in Thailand: a Qualitative Analysis." In B. Yoddumnern-Attig, G.A. Attig, W. Boonchalaksi et al., eds., *Qualitative Methods for Population and Health Research*, 194: 333-344. Bangkok: Insitute for Population and Social Research, Mahodol University.

Quimby, Ernest 1992. "Anthropological Witnessing for African Americans: Power, Responsibility, and Choice in the Age of AIDS." in Gilbert Herdt and Shirley Lindenbaum, eds. *The Time of AIDS.* Newbury Park, CA: Sage Publications.

Quinn, T. 1990. Statement to Thirty-third Annual Meeting of the African Studies Association, Baltimore, MD. Panel on AIDS: Current State of the Epidemic and Treatments, 3 November.

Quinn, T.C.; Mann, J.M.; Curran, J.W. et al. 1986. "AIDS in Africa: An Epidemiologic paradigm. " *Science*. 234 (4770): 955-963.

Ramasubban, R. 1990. "Sexual Behaviour and Conditions of Health Care: Potential Risks for HIV Transmission in India." Paper prepared for the IUSSP Seminar on Anthropological Studies Relevant to HIV Transmission, Sonderborg, November 19-22, 1990.

Reguera, M. Escalona. and Benitez, N. Aguero. 1979. "La Participacion Popular en la Gestion Estatal en Cuba." *Rev. Cub. de Administracion de Salud* 5(3):211.

Rehan, N. 1984. "Knowledge, Attitude and Practice of Family Planning in Hausa Women." *Social Science and Medicine*. 18(10):839-844.

Reid, E. 1994. "Approaching the HIV Epidemic: The Community Response." *AIDS Care*. 6(5):551-557.

Rodriguez, R. 1988. National Director of Epidemiology. Personal Communication, June, 1988.

Romero-Daza, N. 1994. "Multiple Sexual Partners, Migrant Labor, and the Makings for an Epidemic: Knowledge and Beliefs About AIDS Among Women in Highland Lesotho." *Human Organization* 53(2):192-205.

Rosenberg, Charles E. 1962. *The Cholera Years*. Chicago: University of Chicago Press.

Rosenberg, M.J. ; Gollub, E.L. 1992. "Commentary: Methods Women Can Use That May Prevent Sexually Transmitted Disease, Including HIV." *American Journal of Public Health*. 82(11):1473-1478.

Rosner,David and Gerald Markowitz 1991. *Deadly Dust: Silicosis and the Politics of Occupational Disease in Twentieth-Century America*. Princeton, NJ: Princeton University Press.

Rothstein, F.; Blim, M. 1991. *The Global Factory: Anthropological Perspectives*. Bergin and Garvey, New York.

Rushton, J.P.; Bogaert A.F. 1989. "Population Differences in Susceptibility to AIDS: An Evolutionary Analysis." *Social Science and Medicine*. 28 (12): 1211-1220.

Rwandan Red Cross. 1992. *The Orphans of Kigali: a Quantitative and Qualitative Study*. Kigali: Info-AIDS Project, Rwandan Red Cross.

San Juan Star, August 15, 1991:14. Interviews with Dr. Giselda Sanabria and Dr. Juan Carlos de la Concepcion Recach.

Sanchez, S. Epidemiologist, MINSAP, 1988. Personal Communication.

Santana, S. 1987. "The Cuban Health System: Responsiveness to Changing Population Needs and Demands." *World Development*. 15(1): 113-125.

Santana, S. 1990. "Whither Cuban Medicine? Challenges for the Next Generation," in Halebsky, S. and Kirk, J., eds. *Transformation and struggle, Cuba faces the 1990's*. Pp. 251-270. New York: Praeger.

Santana, S.; Faas, L. and Wald K. 1991. "Human Immunodeficiency Virus in Cuba: The Public Health Response of a Third World Country." *International Journal of Health Services*. 21:511-537.

Santos-Ortiz, M. 1990. "Sexualidad Femenina Antes y Despues del SIDA." *Puerto Rican Health Science Journal*. 9(1):33-35.

Saxinger, W.C.; Levine, P.H.; Dean A.G. et al. 1985. "Evidence for Exposure to HTLV-III in Uganda Before 1974." *Science*. 227: 1036-1038.

Scheper-Hughes, Nancy. 1993. " Aids, Public Health and Human Rights in Cuba". *Lancet.* 342 (8877): 965-967.

Schoepf, B. G. 1988a. "Women, AIDS and Economic Crisis in Central Africa." *Canadian Journal of African Studies.* 22(3):625-644.

Schoepf, B.G. 1988b. "AIDS and Society in Central Africa: A View from Zaire," in Norman Miller and Richard C. Rockwell, ed. *AIDS in Africa: The Social and Policy Impact.* pp. 211-235. Lewiston, NY: Edwin Mellen (published in association with the African-Caribbean Institute and the National Council for International Health).

Schoepf, B.G. 1991. "Ethical, Methodological and Political Issues of AIDS Research in Africa." [Review] *Social Science & Medicine.* 33 (7): 749-63.

Schoepf, B.G, 1992a. "AIDS, Sex and Condoms: African Healers and the Reinvention of Tradition in Zaire." in Ralph Bolton and Merril Singer, eds., *Rethinking AIDS Prevention: Cultural Approaches.* Pp: 225-245. Philadelphia: Gordon and Breach Science Publishers.

Schoepf, B. G. 1992b. "Women at Risk: Case Studies from Zaïre, " in G. Herdt and S. Lindenbaum, eds. *The Time of AIDS: Social Analysis, Theory, and Method.* Pp.259-286. Newbury Park, CA: SAGE Publications Inc.

Schoepf, B. G. 1993. "AIDS-Action Research with Women in Kinshasha, Zaire'." *Social Science & Medicine.* 37(11):1401-1413.

Schopper, D.1990. "Research on AIDS Intervention in Developing Countries: State of the Art." *Social Science & Medicine.* 30 (12):1265-1272.

Schopper, D. and Walley, J. 1992. "Care for AIDS Patients in Developing Countries: A Review." *AIDS Care.* 4(1):89-102.

Schuler, S. et al. 1985. "Barriers to Effective Family Planning in Nepal." *Studies in Family Planning.* 16(5):260-270.

Schuster, I. 1981. "Perspectives in Development: The Problem of Nurses and Nursing in Zambia," in N. Nelson, ed. *African Women in the Development Process.* Pp.77-97. London: Cass.

Schwartz, J.S. et al. 1988. "HIV Test Evaluation, Performance and Use." *Journal of the American Medical Association.* 259(17): 2574-2579.

Scrimshaw, S.C. 1973. *Lo de Nosotras: Pudor and Family Planning Clinics in a Latin American City.* New York: International Institute for the Study of Human Reproduction.

Seeley, J.; Kajura, E.; Bachengana, C.; Okong, M.; Wagner, U. and Mulder, D. 1993. "The Extended Family and Support for People with AIDS in a Rural Population in South West Uganda: A Safety Net with Holes?" *AIDSCare.* 5(1):117-122.

Seeley, J.A.; Malamba, S. S.; Nunn, A. J.; Mulder, D. W.; Kengeya-Kayonde, J. F.; and Barton, T. G. 1994. "Socioeconomic Status, Gender, and Risk of HIV-1 Infection in a Rural Community in Southwest Uganda." *Medical Anthropology Quarterly.* 8(1):78-89.

Seeley, J.; Wagner, U.; Mulemwa, J.; Kengeya-Kayondo, J.; and Mulder, D. 1991. "The Development of a Community-Based HIV/AIDS Counseling Service in a Rural Area in Uganda." *AIDS Care.* 3:207-217.

Seidel, G. 1993. "The Competing Discourses of HIV/AIDS in Sub-Saharan Africa: Discourses of Rights and Empowerment vs Discourses of Control and Exclusion." *Social Science & Medicine.* 36(3):175-194.

Serwadda, D; Mugerwa, R.D.; Sewankambo, N.K.; Lwegaba, A.; Carswell, J.W.; Kirya, G.B.;Bayley, A.C.; Downing, R.G.; Tedder, R.S.; Clayden, S.A.; et al., 1985. "'Slim Disease:' A New Disease in Uganda and its Association with HTLV-III Infection." *Lancet.* 2(8460):849-852.

Serwadda, D.; Katongole-Mbidde, E. 1990. "AIDS in Africa: Problems for Research and Researchers." *Lancet.* 335(8693):842-843.

7th Annual International Conference on AIDS, Florence, Italy. 1991. Reported in *New Vision.* June 26, 1991.

Sewankambo, N.K.; Carswell, J.W.; Mugerwa, R.D., et al. 1987. "HIV Infection Through Normal Heterosexual Contact in Uganda." *AIDS.* 1(2): 113-116.

Shedlin, M.G. 1982. *Anthropology and Family Planning: Culturally Appropriate Interventions in a Mexican Community.* Ph.D. Dissertation, Columbia University.

Shedlin, M.G. and Hollerbach, P.E. 1981. "Modern and Traditional Fertility Regulation in a Mexican Community: The Process of Decision Making." *Studies in Family Planning.* 12(6/7):278-296.

Sherris, J.D. and Fox, G. 1985. "Infertility and Sexually Transmitted Disease: a Public Health Challenge." *Population Reports.*, Series L, No. 4, July 1983. (reprinted July 1985).

Shilts, R. 1987. *And The Band Played On.* p. xiv and pp. 3-7. New York: St. Martin's Press.

Shire, C. 1994. "Men Don't Go to the Moon: Language, Space and Masculinities in Zimbabwe," in A. Cornwall and N. Lindisfarne,eds. *Dislocating Masculinities: Comparative Ethnographies.* Pp.147-158.London: Routledge.

Showalter,Elaine 1990. *Sexual Anarchy. Gender and Culture at the Fin de Siecle.* New York: Viking.

Simonsen, J. N.; Plummer, F. A.; Ngugi, E. et al. 1990. "HIV Infection Among Lower Socioeconomic Strata Prostitutes in Nairobi." *AIDS.* 4(2):1 39-144.

Singer, M., Flores C.; Davidson L.; Burke G.; Castillo Z.; Scanlon K.; Rivera, M. 1990. "SIDA: The Economic, Social and Cultural Context Of AIDS among Latinos." *Medical Anthropology Quarterly.*4(10):72-114.

Sittitrai, W.; Sujaritraksa, R.; and Wisuttimak, A. 1989."AIDS Education Materials for Thai Commercial Sex Workers: Preliminary Report." Center for AIDS Research and Education, Science Division, Thai Red Cross Society.

Skin and Allergy News.[Editorial.] 1988. "HIV Origin "a Continuing Mystery": Green Monkey Theory Disputed." *Skin and Allergy News.* January: 28.

Slaughter, Diana T. 1983. "Early Intervention and its Effects on Maternal and Child Development." *Monographs of the Society for Research in Child Development.* 48(4):1-83.

Sokoto Maternal Health Project. 1990. "Report of Planning Activities." Usmanu : Danfodiyo University, Sokoto, and Ministry of Health Sokoto, Report of Maternal Health Project for Prevention of Maternal Mortality, June 1990.

Southall, A.W. 1980. "Social Disorganization in Uganda: Before, During and After Amin." *Journal Of Modern African Studies.* 28:

Spieler, J.M. 1990. "Summary Discussion." (remarks of Dr. Lamptey). In Nancy J. Alexander et al. eds. *Heterosexual Transmission of AIDS.* Pp.419-426. New York: Wiley-Liss.

Standing, H. 1992. "Methodological Issues in Researching Sexual Behaviour in Sub-Saharan Africa." *Social Science & Medicine.* 34(5):475-483.

Standing, H. And M. Kisekka. 1989. *Sexual Behaviour in Sub-Saharan Africa: A Review and Annotated Bibliography.*

Stein, Z. and E. Gollub. 1991. Testimony Submitted to the National Commission on AIDS, Denver, Colorado, June 5, 1991.

Stein, Z.A. 1990. "HIV Prevention: The Need for Methods Women Can Use." *American Journal of Public Health.* 80: 460-462.

Sterry, W.; Marmor, M.; Konrads A. et al. 1983. "Kaposi's Sarcoma, Aplastic Pancytopaenia, and Multiple Infections in a Homosexual" (Cologne, 1976). *Lancet.* 1(8330):924-925.

Stock, R. 1983. "Distance and Utilization of Health Facilities in Rural Nigeria." *Social Science and Medicine.* 17(9):563-570.

Stycos, J.M. 1955. "Birth Control Clinics in Crowded Puerto Rico." In Benjamin D. Paul ed.. *Health, Culture and Community.,* Pp. 189-210. New York: Russell Sage Foundation.

Sukkary-Stolba, S. 1985. "Indigenous Fertility Regulating Methods in Two Egyptian Villages," in Lucile F. Newman, ed., *Women's Medicine: A Cross-Cultural Study of Indigenous Fertility Regulation.* Pp. 78-97. New Brunswick, N.J.: Rutgers University Press.

Susser, I. 1985. "Union Carbide and the Community Surrounding It: The Case of a Community in Puerto Rico." *International Journal of Health Services*, 15(4).

Susser, I. 1991. "Women as Leaders: An Environmental Health Struggle in Puerto Rico," in Frances Abrahamer Rothstein and Michael L. Blim. eds. *Anthropology and the Global Factory : Studies of the New Industrialization in the Late Twentieth Century.* New York: Bergin & Garvey, 1992.

Susser, M.; Watson, W.; Hopper, K. 1989. *Sociology and Medicine.* New York: Oxford University Press.

Tabio, F. Alvarez. 1985. *Comentarios a la Constitucion Socialista.* Havana: Editoria Ciencias Sociales.

Tahzib, F. 1989. " An Initiative on Vesicovaginal Fistula." *Lancet.* 1(8650): 1316-1317.

Terry, H. 1989. "En Beneficio de Todo el Pueblo." *America Latina.* 1: 10-15, Jan., 1989 (Editorial Progreso, Moscu).

Terry, H. 1991. Personal Communication., November, 1991.

Terry, H. et al. 1989. "Programa de control del SIDA." Informe Resumen del Ano 1988 y Acumulado. *Rev. Cub. de Higiene y Epidemiologia* 27(4): 491-503.

Terry, H.; Rodriguez, R. 1988. "Division of Epidemiology", MINSAP. Personal Communication, June, 1988.

Terry, H. and Rodriguez,R. 1988 and 1990. Personal Communication.

Tesh, S. 1986. "Health Education in Cuba." *International Journal of Health Services.* 16(1):87-104. *Teso Newsletter.* 1991: 16.

Tierny, John. 1990. "AIDS in Africa: Experts Study Role of Promiscuous Sex in the Epidemic." *New York Times.* Oct 19 '90: A10.

Torres, L. Monzon et al. 1987. "El Medico de la Familia y su Vinculacion con la Comunidad." *Rev. Cub. de Administracion de Salud.* 13(4).

Treichler, Paula A. 1987: AIDS, Homophobia, and Biomedical Discourse: An Epidemic of Signification. in D.Crimp ed., AIDS, Cultural Analysis, Cultural Activism. Pp. 31-70. Cambridge, MA: MIT Press.

Treichler, Paula A. 1988. "AIDS and HIV Infection in the Third World: A First World Chronicle." in Barbara Kruger and Phil Mariani., eds. *Remaking History.* Seattle: Bay Press.

Trotter, George. 1993. "Some Reflections on a Human Capital Approach to the Analysis of the Impact of AIDS on the South African Economy." In Cross, S. and Whiteside, A. *Facing up to Aids: The Socio-Economic Impact in Southern Africa.* Pp. 391-214. New York: St. Martin's Press.

Turner, C.F.; Miller, H.G.; and Moses, L.E. eds. 1989. *AIDS: Sexual Behavior and Intravenous Drug Use.* Washington, DC: National Academy Press.

Turshen, Meredeth. Forthcoming. 1993. "Trends in the Health Sector with Special Reference to Zimbabwe," in M.R. Carter, J. Cason, and F. Zimmerman, eds. *Rebalancing Market, State and Civil Society for Sustainable Development*. Madison: Wisconsin University Press.

Twumasi, P.A.. 1987. "Traditional Birth Attendant Review Programme in Ghana." Commissioned by Ghana Ministry of Health, October 1987.

Uganda Government. AIDS Control Program 1990 Report.

UK NGO AIDS Consortium for the Third World 1990. "Is AIDS a development Issue?" S. Lucas. ed.. London: The Consortium.

United Nations. 1991. *The World's Women 1970-1990: Trends and Statistics*. New York: United Nations Publications, 1991, Sales No. E.90.XVII.3.

United Nations Development Programme (UNDP). 1993. *Young Women: Silence, Susceptibiity and the HIV Epidemic*. New York: UNDP HIV and Development Programme.

United Nations Economic and Social Commission for Asia and the Pacific (UNESCAP). "Husband-Wife Communication and Practice of Family Planning." *Asia Population Studies Series*, No. 16, Bangkok, 1974:26-27.

USAID. 1990. *HIV Infection and AIDS: A Report to Congress on the USAID Program for Prevention and Control*. Washington, D.C.: U.S. Agency for International Development.

USAID. 1993. *HIV/AIDS: The Evolution of the Pandemic*, the Evolution of the Response. Washington, D.C.: U.S. Agency for International Development.

Vachon, F., J. P. Coulaud, and C. Katlama. 1985. "Epidémiologie Actuelle du Syndrome d'Immunodéficit Acquis en Dehors des Groupes à Risque." *La Presse Médicale*. 14(38):1949-1950.

Van de Walle, Etienne. 1990. "The Social Impact Of AIDS in Sub-Saharan Africa". *The Milbank Quarterly*. 68 (supp.1): 10-32.

Vandepitte, J.; Verwilghen, R.; Zachee P. 1983. "AIDS and Cryptococcosis." (Zaire,1977) [Letter]. *Lancet*. 1(8330): 925-926.

Vella, E.E. 1977. "Marburg Virus Disease." *Hospital Update*. January: 35-41.

Viera, J.; Frank, E.; Spira T.J. et al. 1983. "Acquired Immune Deficiency Syndrome in Haitians." *New England Journal of Medicine*. 308(3):125-129.

Vincent, Joan. 1971. *African Elite: The Big Men of a Small Town*. New York: Columbia University Press.

Vittecoq, D.; Roue, R.T.; Mayaud, C. et al. 1987. "Acquired Immunodeficiency Syndrome After Travelling in Africa: An Epidemiological Study in Seventeen Caucasian Patients." *Lancet*. 1(8533):612-614.

Vlassof, C. 1994. "Gender Inequalities in Health in the Third World: Uncharted Ground." *Social Science & Medicine*. 39(9):1249-1259.

Vos, T. 1994. "Attitudes to Sex and Sexual Behaviour in Rural Matabeleland, Zimbabwe." *AIDS Care*. 6(2):193-203.

Wald, K. 1976. *Los hijos del Che*. Extemporaneos, Mexico, 1986. 21. Constitucion Socialista Cubana. Havana: Ministerio de Justicia.

Wasserheit, J.N. et al. 1989. "The Significance and Scope of Reproductive Tract Infections Among Third World Women." *International Journal of Gynecology and Obstetrics*, Suppl. 3:145-168.

Wasserheit, J.N. 1992. "Epidemiological Synergy. Interrelationships Between Human Immunodeficiency Virus Infection and Other Sexually Transmitted Diseases." [Review] *Sexually Transmitted Diseases*. 19(2): 61-77.

Wasserheit, J.N.; Harris, J.R.; Chakraborty, J.; Kay, B.A. 1989. "Reproductive Tract Infections in a Family Planning Population in Rural Bangladesh." *Studies in Family Planning.* 20(2):69-80.

Watney, Simon. 1989. "Missionary Positions: AIDS, "Africa," and Race." *Differences.* 1(1):83-100.

Wawer, Maria, J. 1994. Personal Communication., August.

Wawer, Maria; Nelson K. Sewankambo, Seth Berkley et al. 1994. "Incidence of HIV-1 Infection in a Rural Area of Uganda." *British Medical Journal.* 308 (6931):171-173.

Webb, D. 1994. "AIDS and the Military: The Case of Namibia." *Analysis Africa.* 4(2):4.

Weekly Topic. 1985. Kampala, 3 Sup.

Weekly Topic. 1986. March 1986.

Weekly Topic. 1991. "Editorial." Sept. 6, 1991.

Weiss, B. 1993. "'Buying Her Grave': Money, Movement and AIDS in North-West Tanzania." *Africa.* 63(1): 19-35.

Weiss, M.G. 1988. "Cultural Models of Diarrheal Illness: Conceptual Framework and Review." *Social Science and Medicine.* 27(1):5-16.

Whaley, J. 1991. "El Programa Cubano Antisida ha Tenido Grandes Logros." La Jornada, Mexico DF Aug. 17.

Whiteside, A. 1993. "The Impact of AIDS on Industry in Zimbabwe," in S. Cross and A. Whiteside, eds. *Facing up to AIDS: The Socio-Economic Impact in Southern Africa.* Pp.217-240. London: Macmillan; New York: St. Martin's Press.

Widy-Wirski, R, S. Berkley, S.Okware et. al. 1988. Evaluation of the WHO Clinical Definition for AIDS in Uganda. *JAMA.* 260: 32866-9.

Williams, G. and Ray, S. 1993. *Work Against AIDS.* London: ActionAid; Nairobi: AMREF.

Wilson, D.; Wilson, C.; Greenspan, R.; Sibanda, P. & Msimanga, S. 1989. "Towards an AIDS information strategy in Zimbabwe." *AIDS Education and Prevention.* 1(2) :96-104.

Winsbury, R. and Whiteside, A. 1994. "The AIDS in Africa Conference, Marrakech - a 12 Page Report: Verdict - a Serious Question of Ethics and Management." *AIDS Analysis Africa.* 4(1):1-12.

WHO. 1990a. *In Point of Fact: The Global AIDS Situation, Updated, June 1990.* World Health Organization, Office of Information, Geneva, Switzerland.

WHO. 1990b. *AIDS Cases Reported to WHO by Country.* 1990. PAHO, Washington, D.C.

WHO. 1990c. "Update: AIDS Cases Reported to Surveillance, Forecasting and Impact Assessment Unit (SFI) Office of Research (RES) Global Programme on AIDS 1 October 1990." Geneva: World Health Organization.

WHO. 1990d. *Weekly Epidemiological Record.* 65(1): 1-2.

WHO. 1992. *Proposed Programme Budget For the Financial Period 1992-1995.* Geneva: World Health Organization.

WHO. 1994a. "African Leaders Back OAU call to Save Children from AIDS." *Global AIDSNews.,* no. 3.

WHO. 1994b. "AIDS and the Worldplace: Signs of Hope from Zimbabwe." *Global AIDSNews.,* 1994 no. 1.

WHO. 1994c. "The Current Global Situation of the HIV/AIDS Pandemic." Global Programme on AIDS 1 July 1994." Geneva: World Health Organization.

WHO. 1994d. "HIV Infections in Africa reach a total of 10 Million, Says the WHO. *AIDS Analysis Africa.,*4(1):4.

WHO. 1994e. "World AIDS Day on 1 December: 'AIDS and the Family,'" Press Release WHO/92, 29 November 1994.

Women's International Network. "Women and Health Summary Facts: Genital and Sexual Mutilation of Females (1)." *News.* Lexington, Maine, no date.

World Health Organization. 1986. "Provisional WHO Clinical Case Definition for AIDS." *Weekly Epidemiological Record.* 51(10):71.

World Health Organization. 1987. "Situation in the WHO European Region as of 31 December 1986." *Epidemiological Record.* 17: 117-124.

World Health Organization. 1988. "Situation in the WHO European Region as of 31 March 1988." *Epidemiological Record.* 63: 201-203.

World Health Organization (WHO). 1989. "WHO Consensus Statement: Sexually Transmitted Diseases as a Risk Factor for HIV Transmission." *Journal of Sex Research.* 26(2):272-275.

World Health Organization. 1990. Consensus Statement from the Consultation on Global Strategies for Coordination of AIDS and STD Control Programmes. Geneva: *World Health Organization.*

World Health Organization/Global Programme on AIDS (WHO/GPA). 1990. *AIDS Prevention: Guidelines for MCH/FP Programme Managers. II. AIDS and Maternal and Child Health.* Geneva: World Health Organization, May 1990, WHO/MCH/GPA/90.2.

Worth, D. 1989. "Sexual Decision-Making and AIDS: Why Condom Promotion among Vulnerable Women is Likely to Fail." *Studies in Family Planning.* 20(6 Part 1):297-307.

Worth, D. 1990. "Minority Women and AIDS: Culture, Race, and Gender." *Culture and AIDS.* 1990: 111-135.

Zabin, L.S. and Clark, Jr, S.D. 1981. "Why the Delay: A Study of Teenage Family Planning Clinic Patients." *Family Planning Perspectives.* 13(5):205-217.

de Zalduondo, B.O.; Msamanga, G.I; and Chen, L.C.: 1989. "AIDS in Africa: Diversity in the Global Panic." *Daedalus.* 118 (3):165-204.

Zarembo, Alan. 1991. "AIDS Vaccine Explained." *New Vision.* 27 April 1991.

Zwi, A.B. and Cabral, A. J. 1993. Editorial: "Reassessing Priorities: Identifying the Determinants of HIV Transmission." *Social Science & Medicine.* 36(5):iii-viii.

About the Book

This book offers detailed ethnographic studies from Africa and the Caribbean to explain AIDS in a global and comparative third-world context. The essays move beyond medical or epidemiological models, explaining the epidemic in its economic, social, political, and historical contexts.

About the Editors
and Contributors

Anne V. Akeroyd is a lecturer in the Centre for Southern African Studies, the Centre for Women's Studies and the Department of Sociology, University of York, England. She took a Ph.D. in social anthropology at University College London. Recent papers include, "Gender, food production and property rights; constraints on women farmers in southern Africa" in *Women, Development and Survival in the Third World*, 1991 and "Personal information and qualitative research data: some practical and ethical problems arising from data protection legislation" in *Using Computers for Qualitative Research*, 1991.

    George C. Bond received his Ph.D. in social anthropology from the London School of Economics and is currently Director of the Institute for African Studies at Columbia University and Professor of Anthropology and Education at Teachers College. He has published extensively on Central Africa and his latest books include The Social Construction of the Past, co-edited with Angela Gilliam and Paths of Violence in Africa, co-edited with Joan Vincent.

    Richard C. Chirimuuta was born in Zimbabwe and now lives in Britain. He studied history, politics and sociology and is co-author of *AIDS, Africa and Racism*.

    Rosalind J. Harrison-Chirimuuta was born in Australia where she attended medical school. She studied tropical medicine at the London School of Hygiene and Tropical Medicine and is now an eye surgeon working for the British National Health Service. She co-author of *AIDS, Africa and Racism*.

    John Kreniske received his Ph.D. in anthropology at Columbia University. He is currently Assistant Professor in the Program for International Studies, at New College, Hofstra University and a Research Associate at the HIV Center of Behavioral and Clinical Sciences, Columbia University. He has conducted research and published articles concerning HIV in Puerto Rico, the Dominican Republic and Thailand.

    Shirley Lindenbaum is Professor of Anthropology and Executive Officer in the Department of Anthropology at the Graduate Center of the City University of New York. She is currently Chair of the American Anthropology Association Commission on AIDS Research and Education and a member of the National Research Council Commission on AIDS Research. Her areas of research have included the study of kuru in Papua New Guinea, cholera in Bangladesh and AIDS in the United States. Among her extensive publications are the path-breaking ethnography, *Kuru Sorcery*, and *The Time of AIDS*, co-edited with Gilbert Herdt.

Maryinez Lyons received her Ph.D in history at UCLA in 1987. Since then she has been a Research Fellow at the Institute of Commonwealth Studies, University of London, as well as Honorary Research Fellow in the Department of Epidemiology and Population Studies, at the London School of Hygiene and Tropical Medicine. She has written numerous articles, the most recent of which is entitled "Foreign Bodies: the History of Labour Migration as a Threat to Public Health in Uganda," Paul Nugent (Ed.), *African Boundaries, Barriers, Conduits and Opportunities*, London: Francis Pinter, 1996. She has also published a book, *The Colonial Disease: Sleeping Sickness in the Early Colonial Belgian Congo, 1890-1940*, Cambridge: Cambridge university Press, 1992.

Regina McNamara is Assistant Professor of the Faculty of Medicine at Columbia University. She has worked on family planning program development in sub-Saharan Africa. Most recently, she has engaged in behavioral research related to the transmission of AIDS and other STDs in Thailand and Uganda.

Elizabeth Reid was one of the main architects of the Australian National AIDS Strategy, probably the first National AIDS Program developed without pressure from a donor agency. Elizabeth is Program Director of the Women and Development Division of UNDP and policy advisor on AIDS and development.

Zena Stein is Professor of Public Health (Epidemiology) at Columbia University, and Associate Dean for Research in the Columbia University School of Public Health, Director of the Epidemiology of Brain Disorders Department of New York State Psychiatric Institute and Co-Director of the HIV Center for Behavioral and Clinical Sciences at Columbia University. She received her medical degree in 1950, from the University of Witwatersrand in Johannesburg, South Africa. Since 1987, she has been co-director of the NIMH-funded HIV Center for Clinical and Behavioral Studies at the New York State Psychiatric Institute and Columbia-Presbyterian Medical Center. She has written extensively on epidemiological issues, with 197 papers and 4 books to her credit. Over the last few years she has spearheaded and led the conceptualization and implementation of Methods Women Can Use in the battle against HIV infection.

Ida Susser received her Ph.D. in anthropology from Columbia University. She is currently Professor of Anthropology at Hunter College and in the Doctoral Program of Anthropology at the Graduate Center for the City University of New York. She is the Director of the International Anthropology of AIDS Group in the HIV Center for Behavioral and Clinical Sciences, Columbia University, which included all the editors of this book. She has conducted research with respect to health and HIV prevention in New York City, Puerto Rico and South Africa and in addition to her book, *Norman Street: Poverty and Politics in an Urban Neighborhood*, has published numerous articles concerning issues of poverty, gender and political mobilization.

Meredeth Turshen received her Ph.D from the University of Sussex. After twelve years experience working with UNICEF of the United Nations, she joined the faculty of Rutgers University. She is currently Associate Professor in the Edward J. Bloustein School of Planning and Public Policy there. She has published extensively on problems of health in Africa and is currently working on a book, to be called *The Demise of Health in Africa: Implications for Gender Equity.*

Joan Vincent received her Ph.D. from Columbia University and is currently Professor Emeritus of the Department of Anthropology, Barnard College. Her research has been in Africa and Northern Ireland and she has published extensively concerning the historical emergence of political conflict and ethnicity. Her most recent books are *Anthropology and Politics* and the *Paths of Violence in Africa*, co-edited with George Bond.

Index